THE ESSENTIAL GUIDE TO AT-HOME TRAINING

Matt Brzycki

a RAM Publishing Production
Blue River Press
Indianapolis, Indiana

LCCN:

Printed in the United States of America
10 9 8 7 6 5 4 3 2 1

Published in the United States by
Blue River Presss
Indianapolis, Indiana 46264

ACKNOWLEDGEMENTS

Even though the name of one author may appear on the cover, a book is never really done by one person. A sincere thanks to . . .

Mark Collins of Bright Ideas Graphics for designing a truly exceptional cover.

Holly Kondras who did the layout and design of the text and coordinated the production of the book.

Tony Alexander who offered suggestions on the content of the first chapter and reviewed the manuscript prior to publication.

Fred Fornicola who was quick to offer his assistance in taking and editing more than 100 photographs for the book.

Ray Abayon, Tony Alexander, Charity Bonfiglio, Ryan Bonfiglio, Alicia Brzycki, Ryan Brzycki, Jennifer Caissie, John Caissie, Fred Fornicola, Lori Fornicola, Lucian Grimaldi, Benjamin Hart, Robert Hilkert, Nicole Meyer, Tara Meyer, Wayne Meyer, Tom O'Rourke, Adam Re, Doug Scott, Joe Siciliano and Pete Silletti for providing the pictures that appear in this book and/or volunteering their time to pose for the pictures.

Rhonda Johnson who offered the use of her camera in order to take several last-minute photographs.

Precor, Incorporated, for providing two photographs that appear in Chapter 2.

Cybex International, Incorporated, for providing the artwork that appears in Appendices A and B.

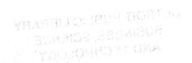

To my wife, Alicia, and our son, Ryan

Other books by Matt Brzycki:

- *The Female Athlete: Reach for Victory* (co-author)
- *Wrestling Strength: Dare to Excel*
- *The Female Athlete: Train for Success* (co-author)
- *Conditioning for Baseball* (co-author)
- *SWAT Fitness* (co-author)
- *Wrestling Strength: Prepare to Win*
- *Wrestling Strength: The Competitive Edge*
- *Maximize Your Training* (editor)
- *Cross Training for Fitness*
- *Youth Strength and Conditioning*
- *A Practical Approach to Strength Training*
- *Conditioning for Basketball* (co-author)

TABLE OF CONTENTS

A Few Words of Caution:

While you're to be commended for your enormous enthusiasm about at-home training, you should be aware of the potential risks of exercising (at home or elsewhere). It's important to know that the following individuals should receive medical clearance from a physician before beginning an exercise program: older adults (men who are 45 or more and women who are 55 or more); those who are at a high risk for cardiovascular disease (such as those who are sedentary or obese or have high blood pressure, high cholesterol or a history of cardiovascular disease in their families); and those who have cardiac, pulmonary or metabolic disease.

1

THERE'S NO PLACE LIKE HOME!

Like virtually everything else, at-home training has advantages as well as disadvantages. But with a little creative effort, even the disadvantages can be overcome.

ADVANTAGES

There are many advantages of at-home training. For one thing, you don't have to sign any contracts or pay "initiation" fees or monthly dues. In addition, you won't have to waste time by driving to the gym. Nor will you waste any time looking for – or worrying about – a parking space. Needless to say, you won't have to wait in line for equipment when training in the comfort of your home. Moreover, you can listen to whatever type of music that you desire – or you can choose not to listen to any music whatsoever. You don't have to worry about when the gym opens or closes – you can train whenever you want! Finally, you won't have to experience any of the distractions that are associated with commercial gyms such as having to deal with obnoxious members.

DISADVANTAGES AND COUNTERMEASURES

Unfortunately, at-home training has the potential for several disadvantages. The good news is that not all of the disadvantages may be relevant to you. And often, those that are relevant can be countered effectively. Let's look at several of the more common disadvantages that can affect most people and explore some tactics to overcome them.

Photo 1-1: Needless to say, you won't have to wait in line for equipment when training in the comfort of your home.

Staying Motivated

One potential drawback of at-home training is staying motivated. Though this can occur in a commercial gym, it's more likely to occur in a home gym. Clearly, a lack/loss of motivation can be very difficult to resolve. One suggestion for dealing with this dilemma is setting short-term goals that are reasonable and attainable. Some people fall into the trap of setting a long-term goal that's unreasonable and well beyond their means. While this approach may sound admirable, it's often destined to failure. For example, an individual might have this thought: "I

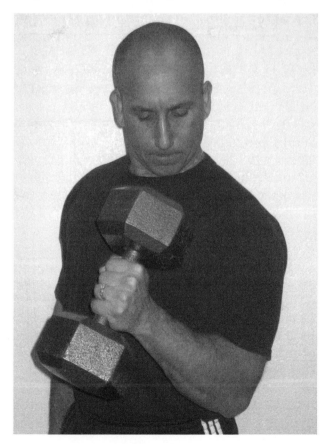

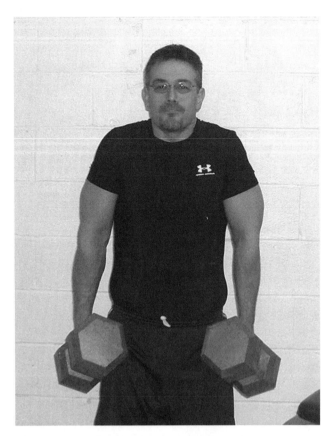

that you do while strength training and conditioning. (This concept will be explored in more detail in subsequent chapters.)

Limited Equipment

For many people, another potential disadvantage of at-home training is having a limited amount of equipment – which may be the result of either cost or space. For instance, you might not be able to afford a leg curl/extension machine or have sufficient room to install one in your home. And how many times have you heard or thought, "If I just had *that* piece of equipment, I'd really be able to get in top shape." Sure, having particular pieces of equipment can make it easier to address specific muscles or perform certain activities. But not having access to particular pieces of equipment shouldn't be a deterrent to starting or continuing a workout program. Remember, too, that people who have equipment in their homes also need to know how to use it properly. Indeed, you could own a Porsche GT2 but it won't do you much good unless you know how to drive a car. While nothing can replace personal instruction from a knowledgeable fitness professional, this book will provide you with the next best thing: a substantial base of knowledge to perform exercises in a safe and productive fashion.

The fact is that even if you don't have *any* exercise equipment, you can still design a fairly comprehensive workout that you can do without having to join a commercial gym. Your routines can start out by simply doing just a few activities or exercises that will elevate your heart rate to an appropriate level. For example, one of the best activities that you can do is walking; it's natural, inexpensive and can be done just about anywhere. (Though not a necessity, you can invest a few dollars in a pedometer which is a device that will count your steps. Some pedometers can be programmed for your specific stride length and bodyweight and then use this information to estimate mileage and caloric expenditure. Your goal should be to walk at least 10,000 steps a day which – based upon a 32-inch stride on a

remember that I used to be able to run a seven-minute mile. So, there's no reason why I can't do that again within the next month or so." While the intent is well meaning, what if the individual hasn't run or done any kind of significant activity in years? Well, this is what's likely to happen: The person attempts to run too far too quickly, ends up getting hurt or excruciatingly sore, loses motivation and, in frustration, quits the conditioning program. The same thing often happens when someone initiates a strength-training program: The individual attempts to use a resistance that's too heavy or uses too much volume, gets hurt or is in a great deal of pain for days, loses motivation and stops lifting weights.

Setting short-term, reasonable goals is a simple yet effective solution to this problem. This will help you to decrease your chances of injury, ensure that your enthusiasm will endure and increase the likelihood of your adherence to a workout program. Feeling the accomplishment of reaching a pre-determined goal can do wonders for your psyche. And while on the subject of motivation, let's not forget the importance of keeping some sort of log of your performances. In brief, you should keep a record of everything

Photo 1-3: An inexpensive investment that will add numerous movements to your inventory of exercises in a resistance band/cord.

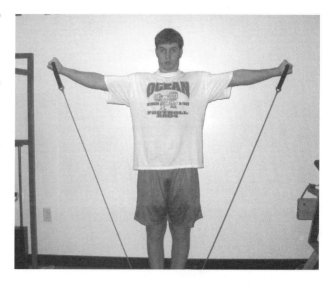

level surface – is a little more than five miles.)

Also not requiring any equipment are several bodyweight or calisthenic-type exercises such as push-ups and crunches. And, of course, you don't need any equipment to do stretching movements. Certainly, doing any of these activities/exercises is much better than doing nothing at all. Having said that, an inexpensive investment that will add numerous movements to your inventory of exercises is a resistance band/cord. So, there are many more options than you might think for at-home training with a limited amount of equipment, space and money.

Domestic Distractions

The atmosphere of training in your home may produce distractions that are unlike those that might be found in a commercial gym – and some of them may be difficult to overcome. It's so easy to interrupt, postpone or even abandon a workout when there are other projects and chores around the house that require your attention. Phone calls and doorbells; house work and yard work; significant others and children. These and other obstacles have the potential to become formidable deterrents to at-home training. Think about it: Do you answer the doorbell or lift the dumbbell? How, then, do you counter these and other distractions? In general, try to stay focused as much as possible on your primary goal: to complete your workout as planned. Workouts of relatively brief duration – by the very nature of the low involvement of time – can help you to maintain your focus.

Time Commitment

Finding the time to work out can be another disadvantage. However, this is actually an *advantage* of at-home training. If you train at home, you won't waste precious time fighting traffic on the way to (and from) the gym, looking for a place to park your Porsche GT2, standing in line waiting to use your favorite piece of equipment and so on. Finding the time to work out has al-

ways been a critical part of the thought process. "What time do I have to work out? Maybe I could do it in the morning? Or maybe I could do it in the evening? I wonder if I could squeeze it in during lunchtime? But I just don't have enough time!" Well, the truth is that we all have at least *some* time. So, the real issue isn't *having* time; rather, it's a matter of *making* time.

If you do have legitimate time constraints, there's still hope. According to the American College of Sports Medicine, an individual should exercise 3 - 5 times per week for 20 - 60 minutes to improve aerobic (or cardiovascular) fitness. But the 20 - 60 minutes doesn't have to be continuous – it can be distributed throughout the day. So if you don't have a one-hour block of time available, you can divide your workout into several smaller sessions. Look at it this way: You can obtain 60 minutes of activity by doing one session that lasts 60 minutes, two sessions that last 30 minutes each, three sessions that last 20 minutes each or even four sessions that last 15 minutes each. And as mentioned earlier, brief workouts can help you to keep your focus on the objective at hand.

HOME SWEET HOME

Your task is to weigh the advantages and the disadvantages of at-home training to determine whether or not you can obtain a safe and productive workout without having to join a commercial gym. When the dust settles, you may discover that there's no place like home!

2
EQUIPPING YOUR HOME GYM

As noted in Chapter 1, you can perform a reasonably comprehensive workout without having access to any equipment. Most people, however, invest in at least some equipment. While many people have spent fairly large sums of money on home equipment, a modest investment is often all that's needed.

The two main categories that will be discussed are aerobic (or "cardio") equipment and strength equipment. Several other miscellaneous items will also be noted. The intent of this information is to provide you with general suggestions for making your selections as well as a working knowledge of the advantages and disadvantages of different types of equipment. However, specific equipment will not be recommended – or, for that matter, even mentioned – and specific manufacturers will not be endorsed. For recommendations on particular pieces of equipment, you're encouraged to consult buyer-friendly publications such as *Consumer Reports* and *Consumers Digest*.

When making decisions about purchasing equipment, you should consider certain things. Here are some general suggestions:

- Stay away from cheap products. As they say, "You get what you pay for." This statement is especially true of exercise equipment. You should buy products that are made by reputable manufacturers that have a proven track record. Look at it this way: There's a good chance that the money you save on purchasing low-cost equipment will eventually be spent on making high-cost repairs.

- Consider low-end commercial equipment. Sometimes, there's not much of a price difference between high-end residential equipment and low-end commercial equipment. Besides, the added durability of a commercial-grade product may compensate for its extra cost.

- Research the equipment before you go to a dealer. This way, you'll be more knowledgeable about the equipment and have a better understanding of how it functions and what it costs.

- Give it a try before you buy. You wouldn't want to purchase an automobile without first taking it for a spin, would you? Most dealers have showrooms where you can "test drive" equipment. And when you do try it out, take your time.

- Buy equipment that you'll use. For instance, don't purchase a stationary bicycle if you don't enjoy cycling. In all likelihood, it'll end up collecting dust in a desolate area of your home.

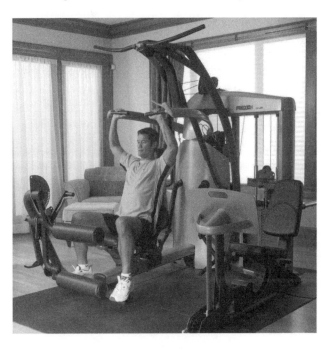

Photo 2-1: You should buy products that are made by reputable manufacturers that have a proven track record.

- Get detailed information about the warranty. Find out what's covered. Is it a bumper-to-bumper warranty? In other words, are the frame and all of the parts covered? If so, how long? Is labor included in the warranty? If so, how long?

- Find out exactly what happens if the equipment needs to be repaired. For example, is the dealer responsible for contacting the manufacturer to obtain a repair part or is that up to you? The part might be under warranty but who actually makes the repair? Does the dealer send one of its technicians to your home or is the onus on you?

- Clarify the return policy. At what point are you no longer eligible for a full refund?

- Shop around. Get specifics on the equipment that you want to purchase and visit other dealers to evaluate their prices and warranties. But make sure that you compare apples to apples. For instance, don't simply compare the price of a treadmill that's made by one manufacturer to that of another without also considering the specifications. Likewise, don't compare different models of a treadmill that are made by the same manufacturer since different models have different specifications.

- Determine if delivery and installation are included in the price. If you have access to a pickup truck and you're handy with tools, you can save some money by doing the delivery and assembly by yourself or with the help of a friend.

- Negotiate expensive purchases. Ask the salesperson, "Is that the best price that you can give me?" If the individual won't budge on the price, perhaps you can make a deal for free delivery, an upgrade or a longer warranty.

AEROBIC EQUIPMENT

This book is meant to assist you with training inside your home. Be that as it may, it would be inappropriate to ignore the convenient and inexpensive aerobic activities that can be done outside your home. As a result, the upcoming discussion will focus upon indoor activities but will also note some outdoor activities.

The following information details the most popular and effective equipment for aerobic training that's currently available. Included is a candid discussion of the advantages and disadvantages of each type of equipment.

Cross-Country Ski Machines

Exercising on a cross-country ski machine is a productive way to improve your aerobic fitness without subjecting your body to high-impact forces. Another advantage is that it demands the coordinated efforts of virtually all of your major muscle groups. Because it influences such a large amount of muscle mass, your caloric expenditure can be very high (though this depends upon your level of intensity). A disadvantage is that it demands some degree of proficiency and coordination.

With some machines, the motion of the skis is dependent-action – the movement of one ski acts counter to the movement of the other ski. In other words, as one ski moves forward, the other ski moves backward the same distance. On other models, the skis move independently – each ski functions separately from the other. (Helpful hint: Look for an independent-action machine since it provides a more realistic way to "ski.")

Obviously, cross-country skiing also can be performed outdoors. Like its indoor counterpart, doing it outdoors addresses an extensive amount of muscle mass. On the downside, cross-country skiing can be expensive. It also requires proficiency and coordination – even more than the indoor version. Another drawback is that it's a seasonal activity that requires snowy surroundings.

Elliptical Machines

The first elliptical machine of any meaningful value was unveiled in 1995. (The term "elliptical" refers to the pattern that the pedals make when the machine is viewed from the side.) Since then, it has become an increasingly popular piece of equipment for aerobic training. The likely reason for the widespread appeal of an elliptical machine – or, simply, "elliptical" – is that it lets you perform an effective, no-impact activity with a relatively low level of perceived exertion. Many ellipticals have an upper-body component that allows you to address all of your major muscles groups, not just those in your hips and legs. This means that you can use a considerable amount of calories. A disadvantage of an elliptical is that a quality one is usually expensive. Another drawback is that it takes up a good deal of space.

Exercise/Fitness Videos

Exercising with a video can be an effective way of increasing aerobic fitness. There are literally hundreds of exercise/fitness videos that are available on a wide range of topics including yoga, pilates, tai chi, kickboxing (and other "combative" variants), floor aerobics, step aerobics and aqua aerobics. Some exercise/fitness videos involve the use of hand-held weights or a resistance band/cord; others focus entirely upon specific muscle groups such as the hips and abdominals. There are even videos for stretching and strength training with free weights and machines. (Helpful hint: Look for videos that are appropriate for your level of fitness.)

Using a video has a number of appealing features. If the video happens to include music, it makes the activity more enjoyable. The person or "instructor" in the video can provide motivation – almost as if you're not exercising alone. If you exercise with the same video too many times, however, monotony can rear its ugly head. But as noted earlier, a wide selection of videos is available which reduces the possibility of boredom.

There are several other drawbacks with exercise/fitness videos. Many of the videos require a certain level of skill and coordination which may be a problem for some people, especially beginners. A major concern that's specific to some of the videos is the potential for chronic and acute injuries. Over the course of time, for example, doing high-impact aerobics can place an inordinate amount of stress on the ankles, knees and lower back. These orthopedic demands can quickly lead to a variety of overuse injuries. Low-impact aerobics – that is, keeping at least one foot on the ground at all times – reduces the amount of orthopedic stress and is a favorable alternative. The flooring is a very important factor in reducing the risk of injury: The softer and more yielding the surface, the less orthopedic stress on your bones, joints and connective tissues. Along these lines, appropriate footwear that provides plenty of cushion, support, flexibility and traction should also be worn.

Photo 2-2: The eliptical machine has become an increasingly popular piece of equipment for aerobic training.

Jump Ropes

There are a few advantages of using a jump rope to improve your aerobic fitness. Rope jumping is inexpensive, portable, requires very little space and can be performed just about anywhere. (Helpful hint: Look for a rope that has handles containing ball bearings – this makes the effort easier and smoother.)

Rope jumping does have a few drawbacks. In order to produce adequate benefits, you must have a fair amount of proficiency at jumping rope. Some people may need a considerable amount of practice in order to master the skill. Although rope jumping will exercise your upper and lower bodies simultaneously, a relatively small amount of muscle mass – your calves and forearms – often receives much of the workload. But the biggest disadvantage of rope jumping is that it's an extremely high-impact activity. Compared to low-impact activities, jumping rope has a much higher risk of excessive orthopedic stress – particularly to the ankles, knees and lower back – and a greater potential for overuse injuries. To reduce the risk, you should jump rope on a soft, yielding surface and use good footwear that has adequate cushion and support in order to help absorb the impact.

Rowing Machines

The coordinated efforts of nearly all of your major muscle groups are involved in rowing: your hips, legs, lower back and the pulling muscles of

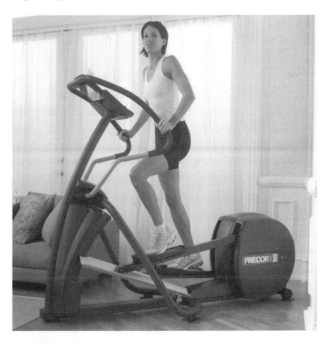

your torso. Exercising continuously with this large amount of muscle mass can create a sizable expenditure of calories. (Helpful hint: Look for a rowing machine – or "rower" – that gives a true simulation or feeling of actually pulling an oar through water.)

Some rowing machines take up a good bit of space but many are portable. Here's a disadvantage: Since the lower back is used a great deal in rowing, those with low-back problems will have a difficult time exercising in a pain-free manner. Another downside is that rowing requires a large degree of technique. Using proper technique is especially important so that you obtain maximum benefits and reduce your risk of injury. (Training tip: Begin the "drive" phase of the rowing movement by extending your hips, legs and lower back and finish the stroke by pulling the handle to your mid-section with your arms. At the end of the stroke, your legs should be straight and you should be leaning slightly backward. The "recovery" phase is done in the reverse order, starting by straightening your arms and then bringing your torso forward while flexing your hips and legs.)

Rowing, of course, also can be done outdoors. A disadvantage of outdoor rowing is the need for a body of water that's accessible and suitable for rowing. Like other outdoor activities, the weather also can present a problem. Finally, the equipment can be rather expensive.

Stairclimbers/Steppers

In 1984, the era of stairclimbers/steppers began at a Chicago trade show in a vendor booth that measured a meager 8 x 10 feet. Despite this rather anonymous and humble beginning, these machines have grown increasingly popular. In general, a stairclimber/stepper features two steps on which you stand and exercise. There are two categories of "two-step" models: dependent and independent. With a dependent-action stairclimber/stepper, the movement of one step is counter to the movement of the other step. In other words, as one step goes down a certain distance, the other automatically comes up the same distance. With an independent-action stairclimber/stepper, each step operates separately from the other. (Helpful hint: Look for an independent-action machine since it makes stepping feel more natural.)

When used correctly, a stairclimber/stepper can be extremely productive and physically demanding. It's fairly easy to operate and provides low-impact activity since your feet never leave the steps. A few machines also provide activity for the muscles of your torso which can increase your caloric expenditure.

On the downside, many stairclimbers/steppers are of poor quality and may not be very durable. A quality machine can also be quite expensive. Another disadvantage of a stairclimber/stepper is that you must utilize proper technique to get maximum benefits. (Training tip: Avoid supporting your body on the handrails or the front of the machine.) Most importantly, however, is the fact that some stairclimbers/steppers are poorly designed and may predispose the knees to hyperextension at the bottom portion of the movement. In particular, the knees are exposed to high levels of orthopedic stress when using dependent-action stairclimbers/steppers. The safest machines are the ones in which the surface of the steps remain parallel to the floor throughout their travel.

An effective alternative that's closely related to mechanical stairclimbers/steppers is bench stepping. This can be done in your home by simply climbing up and down a staircase or stepping up on and down from several aerobic steps stacked on the floor. The outdoor equivalent of indoor bench stepping is walking up and down the steps at a public stadium. A disadvantage of bench stepping is that it's a high-impact activity because your feet leave the ground thereby increasing the potential for injury. Another disadvantage of bench stepping is the distinct potential for boredom.

Stationary Bicycles

One of the most widely used pieces of exercise equipment is the stationary bicycle or "bike." Exercising with a stationary bicycle has several advantages. For starters, it's inexpensive and easy to use – no balance, coordination or special skills are needed. A stationary bicycle is portable and takes up very little space. In addition, you can target the muscles of your lower body in an effective manner without any impact forces. Furthermore, some stationary bicycles give you the option of doing activity just for your torso. This is advantageous for several reasons. In the event

Photo 2-3: Some stationary bicycles give you the option of doing activity just for your torso.

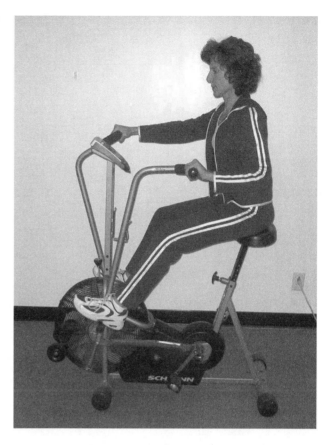

of an injury to your lower body, you still can continue your aerobic training. It also offers increased variety: You can exercise with just your legs, just your arms or both your arms and your legs.

A welcome innovation that has quickly gained favor among fitness enthusiasts is the recumbent bicycle. When using this particular machine, you're positioned in a wide, car-like, bucket seat with your feet in front of you (rather than underneath you). Compared to an upright position, a recumbent position enhances comfort dramatically and reduces the stress on the lumbar spine.

Bicycling also can be done outdoors. In fact, it was probably one of the first outdoor activities that you ever learned as a child. Outdoor bicycling is fairly inexpensive and, for variety, can be done over different terrains ranging from neighborhood streets to various roads and trails. For some people, a drawback of outdoor cycling is that it requires more balance and coordination than its indoor counterpart. Outdoor cycling also carries with it a relatively small but ever-present risk of injury. Regardless of the local laws, it's a good idea for you to wear protective apparel – especially headgear.

Swimming/Aquatic Exercising

Several aquatic activities can be done in the shallow end of the pool such as calisthenics and aqua aerobics as well as walking, jogging and running through the water. But the most popular of all aquatic activities is swimming.

There are many advantages of doing activities in a pool. For one thing, many water-based activities – particularly swimming – involve the collective efforts of your upper- and lower-body muscles. This large amount of musculature can require a high level of caloric expenditure. More importantly, activities that are done in an aquatic environment are non-weightbearing which eliminates the impact forces on your bones, joints and connective tissues. Since the water supports your bodyweight, aquatic activities have a lower potential for musculoskeletal injuries than traditional weightbearing activities.

An obvious drawback is that you must have access to a swimming pool. A disadvantage of aquatic activities is that some individuals may not be comfortable in water. There are several other downsides that are specific to swimming. In order to produce maximum benefits, you must possess a fair level of proficiency at swimming. Some people may need a considerable amount of practice in order to master the skill. If you aren't skilled at swimming, you'll also tire very quickly. Flotation devices – such as an aqua-vest or a simple kick-board – may help someone overcome any shortcomings of swimming skills.

By the way, the heart-rate response while swimming at a specific oxygen intake is about 14 beats per minute lower than running at the same level of oxygen intake. So, the heart-rate training zone should be slightly lower during swimming compared to other aerobic activities.

Treadmills

Believe it or not, the first treadmill – or "tread" – dates all the way back to 1875. But back then, their use wasn't intended for humans. Rather, animals – such as dogs and horses – ran on the treadmills to "power" agricultural ma-

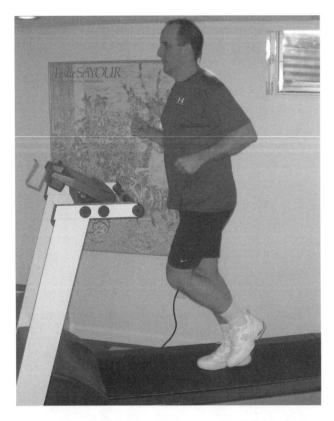

chines. It wasn't until 1952 that the first medical treadmill was invented. And affordable home treadmills weren't sold until the late 1960s. Many years later, one of the most preferred pieces of aerobic equipment is a treadmill.

Basically, there are two types of treadmills: motorized and self-propelled. A motor-driven treadmill tends to be of far better quality than a self-propelled one. There are many advantages of using a treadmill. Walking, jogging or running on a treadmill indoors provides exactly the same aerobic benefits as doing those activities on a track outdoors. Many machines allow you to easily adjust the angle of the deck to either inclined or declined grades which simulates moving uphill or downhill. When using a treadmill, there's no need to worry about uneven surfaces, dangerous traffic, air pollution, exhaust fumes or barking dogs. Finally, many models offer some type of shock-absorbing component beneath the belt that lessens the impact forces. On the downside, a high-quality treadmill is probably the most expensive of all aerobic equipment. Moreover, a treadmill monopolizes a good bit of space.

You can also walk, jog and run outdoors. Besides being simple and natural, doing these activities outdoors doesn't require any special equipment. Another advantage is that you can "change the scenery," so to speak, and avoid the monotony that might occur from using a treadmill indoors while surrounded by the same four walls.

One of the drawbacks of jogging and running is the potential for overuse injuries and other orthopedic problems. There's no question that jogging and running are high-impact activities: It has been estimated that your lower extremities absorb 2 – 3 times your bodyweight when running. So, a person who weighs 170 pounds must dissipate roughly 340 - 510 pounds of impact force with each footfall – and there are more than 1,000 footfalls per mile. The potential for injury is greater when jogging or running on hard surfaces. But jogging or running on a yielding surface such as grass or a treadmill reduces the impact forces.

When jogging or running, it's important to use footwear that's comfortable and durable. Proper footwear also can act as a shock absorber and soften the impact forces. Appropriate footwear should also provide adequate cushion, good heel support and sufficient mid-sole flexibility.

STRENGTH EQUIPMENT

In general, the two most popular types of equipment that are used for strength training are free weights and resistance machines. This is true not only in commercial gyms but also home gyms. What follows is a candid discussion of the advantages of these two types of equipment. (Note: The disadvantages of free weights tend to be the advantages of resistance machines and vice versa. So, discussing the disadvantages of the equipment would be redundant and, therefore, will not be addressed.)

Free Weights

Free weights consist of barbells, weight plates and dumbbells. Here are some advantages of this type of equipment:

• Free weights are generally less expensive than quality at-home machines. And if you're trying to outfit your home gym with a limited or tight budget, this is most important consideration in your choice of equipment. With a bar, adjustable bench and several hundred pounds of plates, you can perform exercises for just about every muscle in your body.

- Free weights can accommodate just about everyone regardless of their size from the largest individual to the smallest. You might say that when it comes to free weights, "one size fits all."

Resistance Machines

Relatively few people have an extensive inventory of commercial-grade, single-station resistance machines in their homes. It's not unusual, though, for fitness enthusiasts to have some type of multi-station apparatus, a cable column (with an adjustable pulley or fixed pulleys in high and low positions) or "home gym" that consists of one or more "stations" at which a number of exercises can be done in a small amount of space. And some of this equipment might not be as expensive as you think. It's these pieces of equipment that will be considered here and discussed elsewhere in this book. Here are some advantages of this type of equipment:

- Resistance machines can make your workouts more time-efficient. You can set the weight on resistance machines by simply moving a selector pin rather than by fiddling around changing plates (unless, of course, it's a plate-loaded machine).

- Resistance machines don't require a spotter. This is true even when lifting a weight over your head – such as during a seated press. Indeed, it's impossible to get pinned underneath a bar or stuck with the weight in a compromising position. (It should be noted that you can do overhead lifting with dumbbells without requiring a spotter for safety.)

- Resistance machines – at least those that are designed properly – automatically vary the weight to match the changes in your biomechanical leverage. In positions of inferior leverage (and inferior strength), the machine creates a mechanical advantage and a lower level of resistance; as your skeletal system moves into a position of superior leverage (and superior strength), the machine creates a mechanical disadvantage and a higher level of resistance. The end result is greater muscular effort throughout the range of motion.

- Resistance machines "balance" the weight for you so that you'll be able to concentrate on the proper performance of the exercise. If the weight isn't balanced, some individuals – particularly those who have very little experience in strength training – might worry more about this aspect than about performing the exercise properly. Furthermore, it's likely that excessive energy will be spent in balancing the weight.

Miscellaneous Items

Finally, there are several items that you also might consider for equipping your home gym. These include the following:

- bench (an adjustable one, if possible)

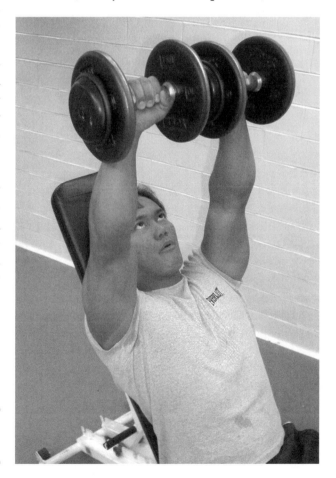

Photo 2-5: You can do overhead lifts with dumbbells without requiring a spotter for safety.

- weight tree (for storing the weight plates)
- EZ-curl bar (in order to perform some exercises)
- dip bars/handles (in order to perform dips and knee-ups)
- chin/pull-up bar (in order to perform chins, pull-ups and knee-ups)
- roller bar (in order to perform wrist rollers)
- attachment ankle/wrist strap, bar and handle (for the cable column)
- wrist straps (to help with your grip on some pulling exercises)
- ankle/wrist weights (for added resistance in some exercises)
- resistance band/cord (in order to perform some exercises)
- stability ball (for variety in your training)

3

STRETCHING YOUR MUSCLES

Flexibility can be defined as "the range of motion (ROM) throughout which your joints can move." The best way for you to maintain – or improve – the ROM of your joints is to perform specific flexibility movements to stretch the surrounding muscles.

Stretching is undoubtedly the simplest and most effortless type of activity that you can do – the exertion level is quite low and relaxation is an absolute requirement. Nevertheless, many people often overlook or underemphasize stretching.

There are a number of reasons why it's a good idea for you to stretch on a regular basis. First, improving your flexibility allows you to move your joints through a greater ROM. Second, being more flexible enables you to exert your strength over a greater ROM. Third, becoming more flexible *may* make you less susceptible to injury. Fourth, stretching your muscles *may* relieve and/or reduce the general muscular soreness that can result from doing unfamiliar activities or intense physical training (although this has yet to be corroborated by research). And think about this: It has been estimated that 80% of the world's population will experience low-back pain sometime in their lives. One contributing factor that's often cited for this problem is a lack of flexibility in the hip flexors and lower back.

FACTORS THAT AFFECT FLEXIBILITY

Your flexibility is influenced by many factors. Generally speaking, there's a distinct relationship between age and flexibility. The greatest increase in flexibility usually occurs up to and between the ages of 7-12. Flexibility tends to plateau during early adolescence and then begins to decline with increasing age. So as you get older, you tend to be less flexible.

Having said that, it appears as if the most significant contributor to decreased flexibility isn't the aging process itself; rather, it's due to a decrease in – or lack of – physical activity. Clearly, then, older individuals can avoid a significant loss of flexibility – and perhaps improve it – by simply being physically active on a consistent basis.

To a degree, your flexibility is also related to your gender. Some men are more flexible than some women but, in general, women are more flexible than men. (Women retain this advantage throughout life.)

In addition, it's important to understand that your flexibility is affected by several genetic (or inherited) factors such as your percentage of body fat (especially that which resides around your mid-section). Your flexibility also has genetic limitations that are structural which include your bones, tendons, ligaments and skin along with the extensibility of your muscles.

As you may already be painfully aware, previous injury to a muscle or connective tissue may also affect your flexibility. Furthermore, immobilizing a joint during rehabilitation may cause the connective tissue to adapt to its shortest functional length thereby reducing the ROM of the joint.

Another factor that influences the flexibility of your joints is your body temperature. Muscles and connective tissues that are warmed up will be more flexible and extensible than muscles and connective tissues that aren't.

Lastly, remember that flexibility is joint-specific – a high degree of flexibility in one joint doesn't necessarily indicate a high degree of flexibility in other joints. So a person who exhibits an adequate level of flexibility in the lower back and hamstrings during a sit-and-reach test, for

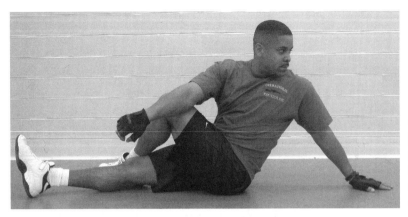

Photo 3-1: It appears as if the most significant contributor to decreased flexibility is a decrease in – or lack of – physical activity

example, may not be flexible in the shoulders and ankles. Along these lines, it wouldn't be uncommon for your flexibility to vary from one side of your body to the other.

WARMING UP

There are two types of warm-ups: passive and active. Passive warm-ups use an external method to increase core temperature (such as hot showers and heating pads); active warm-ups use exercise to achieve this effect (such as light jogging or calisthenics). Surprisingly, the research regarding the need for a warm-up offers conflicting information. Some studies have shown that performances with a prior warm-up are better than those without a warm-up; other studies have shown that performances with a prior warm-up are no different than those without a warm-up. In a few studies, performances actually *worsened* following a warm-up (possibly because the warm-up produced too much fatigue and/or didn't allow sufficient recovery prior to the performance). Nevertheless, a warm-up has both physiological and psychological importance.

Quite often, warming up is viewed as being synonymous with stretching. In reality, however, warming up and stretching are two separate entities and must be treated as such. Warming up the muscles is meant to produce a short-term change to prepare you for an upcoming session of physical activity; stretching the muscles is meant to induce a more long-term change in your ROM.

Warming up should precede stretching. Regardless of the warm-up activity that you choose, the idea is to systematically increase the temperature of your body and the blood flow to your muscles. Breaking a light sweat during the warm-up is a good indication that your core temperature has been raised sufficiently and you're ready to begin stretching your muscles. (When the environmental temperature is high, it's likely that your core temperature is already elevated enough for you to start stretching your muscles.)

As noted previously, muscles and connective tissues that are warmed up have increased flexibility and extensibility. This would mean that biological tissue is most flexible and extensible at the end of a physical activity when your body temperature is elevated. Because of this, some authorities recommend that stretching should be performed *after* you've completed a physical activity. Doing so *may* also relieve and/or reduce general muscular soreness.

By the way, there's no need for you to warm-up or stretch prior to strength training – provided that you perform a relatively high number of repetitions and lift the weight in a deliberate, controlled manner. But it's highly advisable to warm up and stretch prior to a physical activity that involves rapid muscular contractions – such as sprinting – to reduce your risk of injury.

SEVEN STRETCHING STRATEGIES

Though your flexibility may be limited by the factors that were mentioned previously, it can be improved through stretching. Understand that there are two common methods of stretching: static and dynamic. Static stretching is done by easing into a stretch and holding that position; dynamic stretching is done by bouncing repeatedly (and rapidly) in to and out of a stretched position. Static stretching is much safer and more effective than dynamic stretching.

Like all other forms of physical training, stretching has certain guidelines that must be followed in order to make the stretches safe and effective. Adopting these guidelines permits you to maintain or improve your current ROM. Seven strategies for stretching are as follows:

1. Stretch under control without bouncing, bobbing or jerking movements. Bouncing during the stretch actually makes the movement more painful and increases your risk of muscular soreness and tissue damage.

2. Inhale and exhale normally during the stretch without holding your breath. When you hold your breath, it elevates your blood pressure which disrupts your balance and breathing mechanisms.

3. Stretch comfortably in a pain-free manner. Since pain is an indication that you're stretching at or near your structural limits, you should stretch only to the point of mild discomfort.

4. Relax during the stretch. Relaxing mentally and physically allows you to stretch your muscles throughout a greater ROM.

5. Hold the stretched position for about 30 - 60 seconds. Gradually stretching your muscles to a point of mild discomfort, holding that position and then gradually returning them to their pre-stretched state enables you to stretch farther with little risk of pain or injury.

6. Attempt to stretch slightly farther than the last time. Progressively increasing your ROM – and the time that you hold each stretch – improves your flexibility.

7. Perform flexibility movements on a regular basis. You should stretch at least once a day, especially before physical training or any other activity that may involve explosive, ballistic movements.

FLEXIBILITY MOVEMENTS

Similar to other types of training, there's no optimal program for stretching. So, your program can be individualized to suit your personal preferences and special needs. For instance, you may have a greater need to address the flexibility of your hamstrings than someone else.

Fortunately, there are an infinite number of possibilities for designing a stretching program that's comprehensive and effective. Keep in mind that your body has more than 660 muscles. Those muscles influence roughly 200 joints, ranging from those that are relatively immovable (such as the sutures of your skull) to those that are freely movable (such as your hips and elbows). Be that as it may, it isn't necessary to perform a stretch for each muscle. Rather, you simply need to stretch your major muscles. (Remember, too, that most stretches affect more than one muscle.)

You can stretch the muscles that influence your major joints in a comprehensive manner by performing the 16 flexibility movements that are described on the following pages. Included in the discussions of each movement are the muscle(s) stretched, starting position, performance description and training tips for making the movement safer and more effective. (If you need help to identify the muscles, you can refer to the anatomy charts that are shown in Appendices A and B.) The flexibility movements that are described in this chapter are as follows: neck forward, neck backward, lateral neck, scratch back, handcuff, anterior forearm, posterior forearm, standing calf, tibia press, sit-and-reach, V-sit, lateral reach, butterfly, spinal twist, lying quad and knee pull.

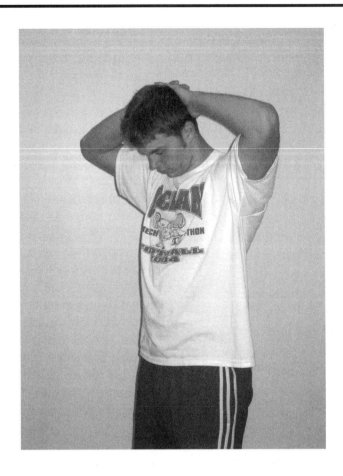

NECK FORWARD

Muscles Stretched: neck extensors and trapezius

Starting Position: While standing, interlock your fingers behind your head.

Performance Description: Slowly pull your chin to your chest.

Training Tips:

- Be especially careful when doing this movement since your cervical area is involved.

- This movement may also be performed while sitting.

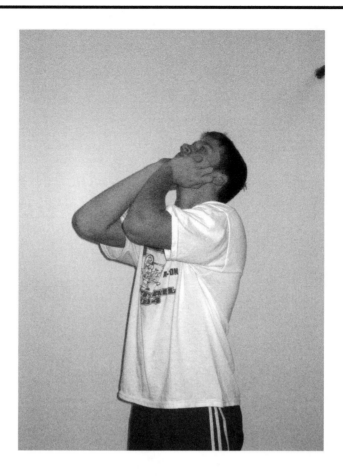

NECK BACKWARD

Muscle Stretched: sternocleidomastoideus (both sides)

Starting Position: While standing, place your hands underneath your chin.

Performance Description: Slowly push your head backward.

Training Tips:

• Be especially careful when doing this movement since your cervical area is involved.

• This movement may also be performed while sitting.

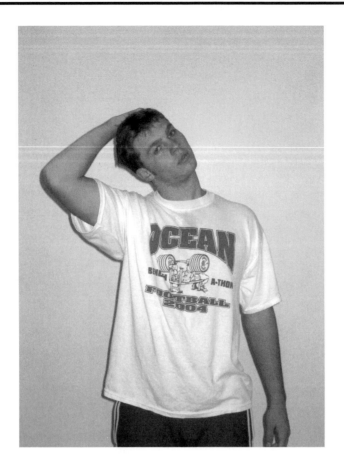

LATERAL NECK

Muscle Stretched: sternocleidomastoideus (one side)

Starting Position: While standing, place your right hand on the left side of your head.

Performance Description: Slowly pull your head to your right shoulder. Repeat the stretch for the other side of your neck.

Training Tips:

- Be especially careful when doing this movement since your cervical area is involved.
- This movement may also be performed while sitting.

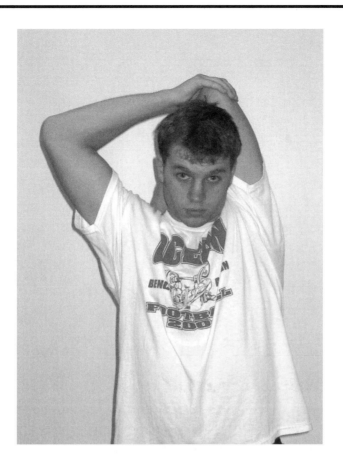

SCRATCH BACK

Muscles Stretched: upper back ("lats"), triceps and obliques

Starting Position: While standing, place your left hand on the upper part of your back (behind your head). Grasp your left elbow with your right hand.

Performance Description: Slowly pull your torso to the right. Repeat the stretch for the other side of your body.

Training Tips:

- For this movement to be most effective, your hips shouldn't move and your feet should remain flat on the floor.
- You should try to gradually reach farther down your back during the stretch.
- This movement may also be performed while sitting.
- This movement may be contraindicated if you have shoulder-impingement syndrome.

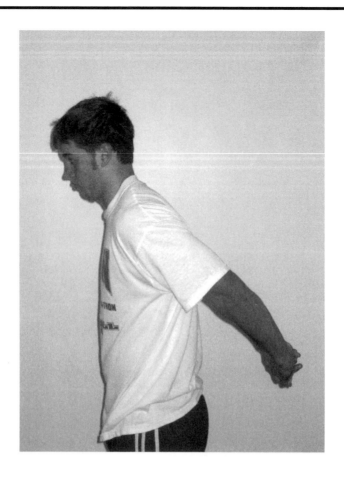

HANDCUFF

Muscles Stretched: chest, anterior deltoid and biceps

Starting Position: While standing, place your hands behind your back and interlock your fingers.

Performance Description: Slowly lift your hands as high as possible.

Training Tips:

- A partner may assist you in obtaining a greater stretch by carefully lifting your hands as you do the movement.
- This movement may also be performed while sitting.

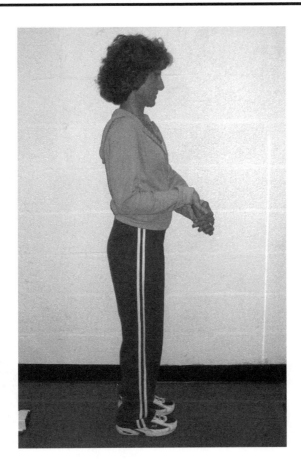

ANTERIOR FOREARM

Muscles Stretched: forearm flexors

Starting Position: While standing, place your right elbow against the right side of your torso and bend your right arm so that the angle between your upper and lower arms is about 90 degrees or less. Point your right palm upward and put your left palm against it.

Performance Description: Slowly push your right hand downward. Repeat the stretch for your other forearm.

Training Tips:

- For this movement to be most effective, you should apply force at a point that isn't too close to your wrist.
- Using one of your hands to pull the other downward will permit a better stretch.
- This movement may also be performed while sitting.

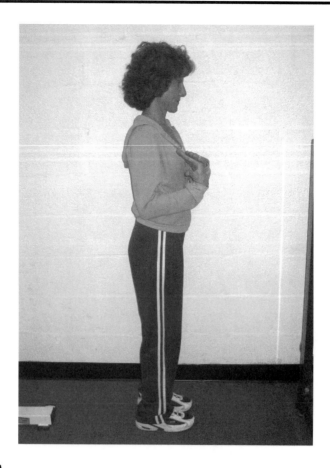

POSTERIOR FOREARM

Muscles Stretched: forearm extensors

Starting Position: While standing, place your right elbow against the right side of your torso and bend your right arm so that the angle between your upper and lower arms is about 90 degrees or less. Point your right palm upward and put your left palm against the back of your right hand.

Performance Description: Slowly push your right hand upward. Repeat the stretch for your other forearm.

Training Tips:

• For this movement to be most effective, you should apply force at a point that isn't too close to your wrist.

• Using one of your hands to push the other upward will permit a better stretch.

• This movement may also be performed while sitting.

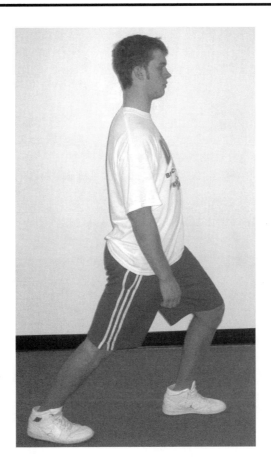

STANDING CALF

Muscles Stretched: calves and iliopsoas

Starting Position: Step forward with your left foot.

Performance Description: Bend your left leg at the knee but keep your right leg straight and your right foot flat on the floor. Repeat the stretch for your other leg.

Training Tip:

- For this movement to be most effective, the heel of your back foot should remain flat on the floor and both of your feet should be pointed forward.

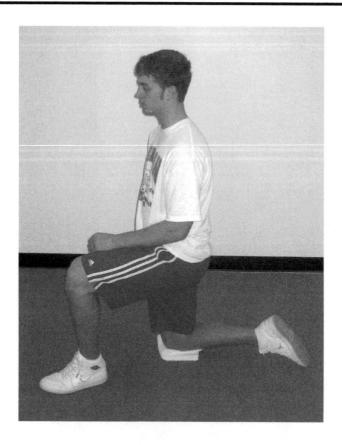

TIBIA PRESS

Muscles Stretched: dorsi flexors

Starting Position: Kneel down on your right knee so that your upper leg is perpendicular to the floor. Position your left leg so that your upper leg is parallel to the floor, your lower leg is perpendicular to the floor and your foot is flat on the floor.

Performance Description: Slowly press your right lower leg and the top part of your right foot flat on the floor. Repeat the stretch for your other leg.

Training Tip:

• For this movement to be most effective, the top part of the foot that's being stretched should be flat on the floor.

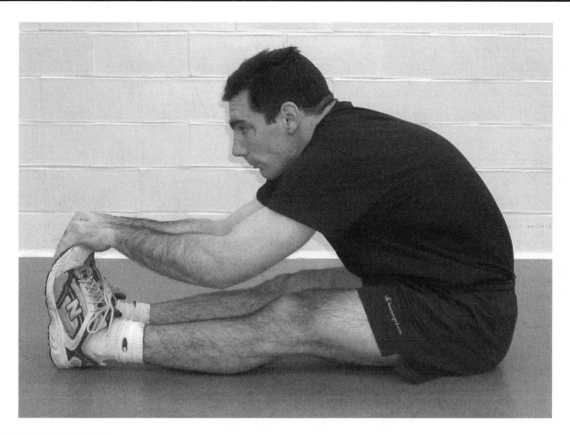

SIT-AND-REACH

Muscles Stretched: gluteus maximus (buttocks), hamstrings, calves, upper back ("lats") and lower back

Starting Position: While sitting, straighten your legs, put them together and point your toes upward.

Performance Description: Without bending your legs, slowly reach forward as far as possible.

Training Tips:

- For this movement to be most effective, your legs should remain straight and your toes should be pointed upward.
- You can progressively stretch farther by reaching for your ankles, your toes and finally your instep.
- A partner may assist you in obtaining a greater stretch by carefully pushing on your upper back as you do the movement.
- This movement may also be performed while standing (with your legs straight and your arms hanging straight down).

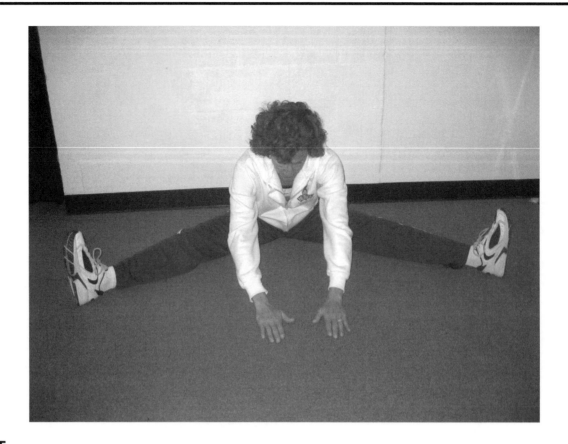

V-SIT

Muscles Stretched: gluteus maximus (buttocks), hip adductors (inner thigh), hamstrings, calves, upper back ("lats") and lower back

Starting Position: While sitting, straighten your legs, spread them apart as far as possible and point your toes upward.

Performance Description: Without bending your legs, slowly reach forward as far as possible.

Training Tips:

- For this movement to be most effective, your legs should remain straight and your toes should be pointed upward.
- You can progressively stretch farther by "walking" your fingers forward.
- A partner may assist you in obtaining a greater stretch by carefully pushing on your upper back as you do the movement.
- This movement may also be performed while standing (with your legs spread apart and your arms hanging straight down).

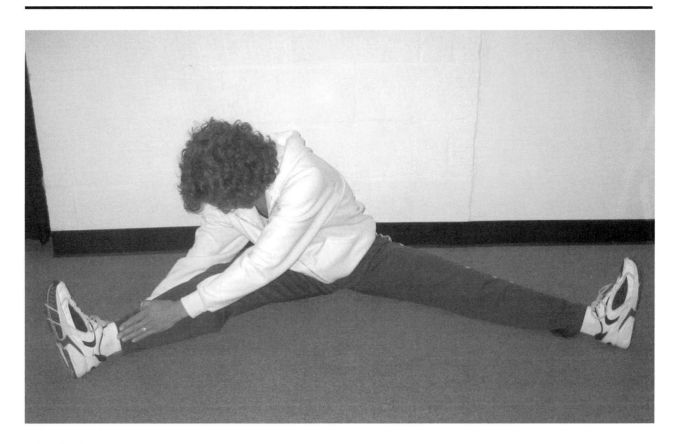

LATERAL REACH

Muscles Stretched: gluteus maximus (buttocks), hip adductors (inner thigh), hamstrings, calves, upper back ("lats"), obliques and lower back

Starting Position: While sitting, straighten your legs, spread them apart as far as possible and point your toes upward.

Performance Description: Without bending your legs, slowly reach down your right leg as far as possible. Repeat the stretch for the other side of your body.

Training Tips:

- For this movement to be most effective, your legs should remain straight and your toes should be pointed upward.
- You can progressively stretch farther by "walking" your fingers forward.
- A partner may assist you in obtaining a greater stretch by carefully pushing on your upper back as you do the movement.
- This movement may also be performed while standing (with your legs spread apart and your arms reaching down your leg).

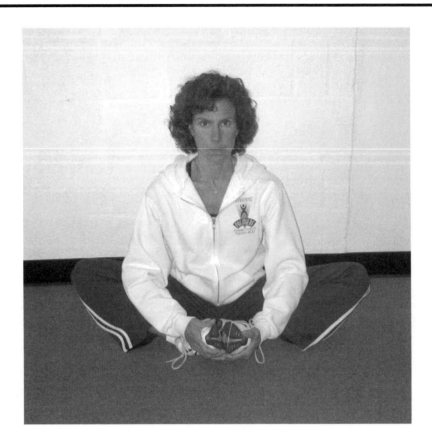

BUTTERFLY

Muscles Stretched: hip adductors (inner thigh) and lower back

Starting Position: While sitting, place the soles of your feet together, draw your heels as close to your body as possible and place your elbows on the insides of your knees.

Performance Description: Bend your torso forward while slowly pushing down with your elbows against the insides of your knees.

Training Tip:

• A partner may assist you in obtaining a greater stretch by carefully pushing on the insides of your knees as you do the movement.

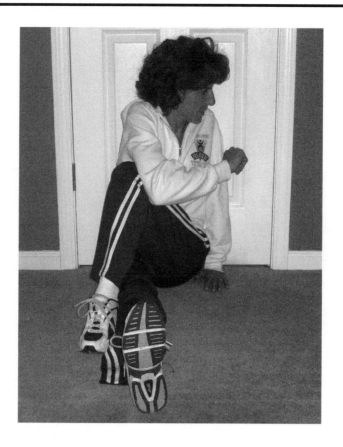

SPINAL TWIST

Muscles Stretched: hip abductors (gluteus medius), obliques and lower back

Starting Position: While sitting, keep your right leg straight, place your left foot on the outside of your right knee and place your right elbow against the outside of your left knee.

Performance Description: Look to your left as far as possible while slowly pushing with your right elbow against the outside of your left knee. Repeat the stretch for the other side of your body.

Training Tip:

- This movement may also be performed while lying supine (by keeping your shoulders flat on the floor and crossing one leg over your body).

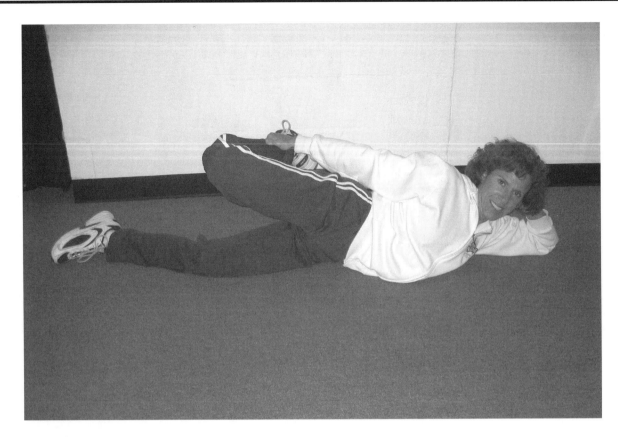

LYING QUAD

Muscles Stretched: quadriceps, iliopsoas and abdominals

Starting Position: Lie on your left side and grasp the top part of your right foot with your right hand.

Performance Description: Slowly pull your right heel toward your buttocks. Repeat the stretch for the other side of your body.

Training Tip:

• This movement may also be performed while lying prone.

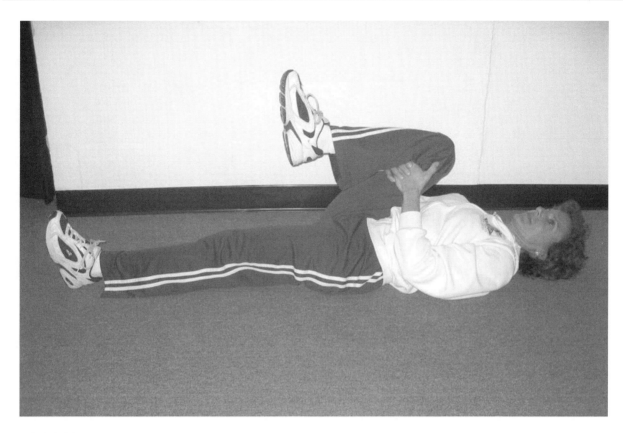

KNEE PULL

Muscles Stretched: gluteus maximus (buttocks), hamstrings and lower back

Starting Position: While lying supine on the floor, straighten your left leg and point your toes upward. Grasp your right leg behind your knee.

Performance Description: Slowly pull your right leg toward your chest. Repeat the stretch for the other side of your body.

Training Tip:

• Using your arms to pull your leg toward your chest will permit a better stretch.

4

IMPROVING YOUR AEROBIC FITNESS

The most important aspect of your physical profile – and the best indicator of your overall health – is your aerobic fitness. Specifically, your aerobic fitness is a measure of how well your muscles consume, transport and utilize oxygen during physical exertions. The best way for you to improve these physiological processes is through aerobic training (which is also known as "cardiovascular training" or, simply, "cardio").

Your aerobic system involves the coordinated efforts of your heart, lungs, blood vessels and other assisting tissues and mechanisms. The main intent of aerobic training is to improve the functional ability of your aerobic system so that it can operate more effectively and more efficiently. This will produce several aerobic benefits including decreased resting and exercising heart rates as well as decreased blood pressure. By improving the functional ability of your aerobic system, you'll also establish a solid foundation of aerobic support for other forms of physical training. Also, a weekend warrior who has a high level of aerobic fitness surrenders to fatigue less quickly than another who has a low level of aerobic fitness – regardless of the sport or activity.

Besides these physiological adaptations, aerobic training – when used in conjunction with sound nutritional practices – helps maintain your percentage of body fat at an acceptable level. And similar to other forms of training, increasing your aerobic fitness will improve many facets of your psychological state such as your self-esteem and self-confidence.

AEROBIC GUIDELINES

Your aerobic fitness may be developed and maintained by implementing several easy-to-follow guidelines that are based upon scientific research. These guidelines can be organized under the acronym "FITT" which stands for "Frequency, Intensity, Time and Type." (Most sedentary individuals can safely begin an exercise program of moderate intensity. However, it's recommended that men at or above the age of 40 and women at or above the age of 50 receive a medi-

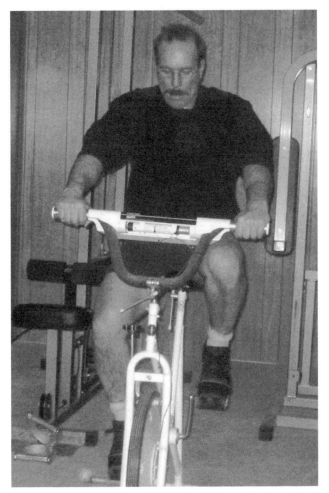

Photo 4-1: To determine an appropriate level of intensity, you should adjust your effort based upon whether the activity feels too easy or too difficult.

cal examination before beginning a vigorous exercise program.)

Frequency

In order for you to improve your aerobic fitness, you need to perform appropriate aerobic activities 3 - 5 days per week. Training less than three days per week doesn't appear adequate enough to promote any meaningful changes in your aerobic fitness; training more than five days per week produces a negligible improvement in your aerobic fitness (which usually isn't worth the time spent).

That being said, training more frequently is beneficial when weight (fat) loss is a goal. But beginning with too much activity too soon may very well lead to an overuse injury such as tendinitis. This is especially true of older individuals as well as those who are inactive or in poor physical condition. People who are susceptible to overuse injuries should initially do aerobic activities 2 - 3 days per week to reduce their potential for orthopedic problems. As these individuals adjust and adapt to the unfamiliar physical demands, they can increase their dosage of aerobic training to 3 - 5 weekly workouts.

Intensity

Other than your inherited characteristics (or genetics), the most important component of your aerobic training is your level of intensity (or effort). Your heart rate increases in direct proportion to the demands of an activity. As such, your training heart rate is commonly used as an estimate of your aerobic intensity. Since there's a slight but steady decrease in your maximal heart rate with aging, estimates of it are made on the basis of your age. In order to receive a benefit from aerobic training it's recommended that you maintain a level of 60 - 90% of your age-predicted maximum heart rate.

One way to find a rough estimate of your age-predicted maximum heart rate in beats per minute (bpm) is to simply subtract your age from 220. For example, the age-predicted maximum heart rate of a 40-year-old individual is 180 bpm [220 - 40 = 180]. To find the recommended heart-rate training zone, multiply 180 bpm by 0.60 and 0.90. This means that a 40-year-old individual needs to maintain a heart rate of about 108 - 162 bpm while training to elicit improvements in aerobic fitness [180 bpm x 0.60 = 108 bpm; 180 bpm x 0.90 = 162 bpm].

Some people may need to maintain their heart rates above the training zone that's recommended for others of the same age. If you're active or have an above-average level of fitness, for example, you should train with a higher percentage of your age-predicted maximum heart rate to receive aerobic benefits; if you're inactive or have a below-average level of fitness, you should train with a lower percentage of your age-predicted maximum heart rate to avoid cardiac risks. Also, you may need to use a lower level of intensity in the early stages of aerobic training to increase the likelihood of your adherence to the program.

Remember, a favorable response depends upon training with an appropriate level of intensity. "Intensity" is a relative term that's determined by each individual's level of fitness. For some people, training with a lower percentage of their age-predicted maximum heart rate may actually represent a high level of intensity and an adequate workload *for them*. Stated otherwise, exercise of low intensity for an active individual may be of high intensity for an inactive individual. Depending upon the initial level of fitness, training with an intensity that's below the suggested range can actually produce some improvement in aerobic fitness.

To determine an appropriate level of intensity, you should adjust your effort based upon whether the activity feels too easy or too difficult. If it feels too easy, increase your intensity; if it feels too difficult, reduce your intensity. Also keep in mind that your intensity – and your heart rate – is influenced by many factors including the environmental conditions (such as the temperature and humidity), your body position (such as being seated or upright) and the amount of muscle mass being trained. (Everything else being equal, training larger muscles will produce a higher heart rate than training smaller ones.)

Your heart rate can be measured easily at several different sites on your body. Numerous heart-rate monitors are available commercially that can give you a reasonably accurate reading of your heart rate. But the easiest and least expensive way to determine your heart rate is to measure it yourself. You can do this by locating your pulse at either the carotid artery (in your neck) or the radial artery (in your wrist). Simply place the tips of your index and middle fingers over one of these sites. Immediately after you complete your aerobic training, count your pulse for 10 seconds. Multiplying that number by six gives you a good estimate of your heart rate while training (in beats per minute). You can obtain a similar estimate by counting your pulse for 15 seconds and multiplying that number by four.

Time

In order for you to improve your aerobic fitness, you should do 20 - 60 minutes of continuous or intermittent activity. ("Intermittent" means that multiple – but briefer – sessions can be done on the same day. As an example, two 15-minute workouts in one day would equal 30 minutes of aerobic activity.) Keep in mind, too, that the time of the activity is inversely proportional to the intensity of the activity. So, the length of your effort can be relatively brief provided that your level of effort is relatively high. In fact, research has shown that training for as little as 10 - 15 minutes can significantly increase your aerobic fitness. But a workout this brief would have to be extremely intense in order to obtain the desired benefit. Generally speaking, investing 20 minutes of continuous or intermittent activity with an appropriate level of effort is enough to improve your aerobic fitness.

It should also be noted that if the length of your aerobic effort is too brief, your workout might not produce a desirable expenditure of calories. This may be an important consideration if one of your primary objectives is to lose weight (fat). In this case, you should perform aerobic activities for at least 30 minutes but no more than 60. (Guidelines for a safe and effective weight-management program are detailed in Chapter 19.)

When your intensity is low – for whatever reason – your activities should be conducted for a longer period of time. Take into account, though, that lengthy workouts may be inappropriate for some people in the initial stages of aerobic training. For one thing, performing too much activity too soon increases the risk of incurring an overuse injury. For another, some individuals may initially have such low levels of fitness that they may only be able to tolerate 5 - 10 minutes of aerobic training. In either case, they can gradually increase the length of their aerobic workouts as they improve their levels of fitness.

Type

The combined application of the aforementioned guidelines concerning the frequency, intensity and duration of aerobic training provides a meaningful workload for your aerobic system. If these three ingredients of aerobic training produce the same expenditure of total calories, your physiological adaptations will be similar regardless of the aerobic activity that you perform. Therefore, you can use a variety of activities to increase your aerobic fitness.

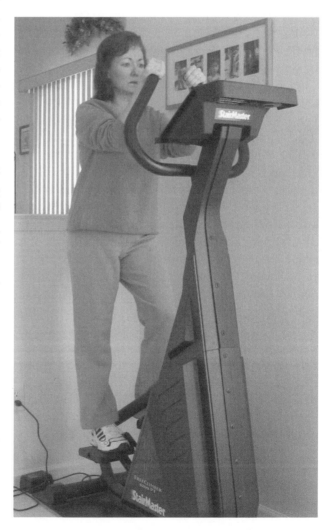

Photo 4-2: In order for you to improve your aerobic fitness, you should do 20 - 60 minutes of continuous or intermittent activity.

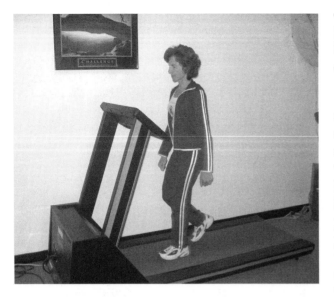

Photo 4-3: You can use a variety of activities to increase your aerobic fitness.

The preferred types of aerobic activities are those that require a continuous effort, are rhythmic in nature and involve large amounts of muscle mass. Popular indoor activities that can be used to stimulate aerobic fitness include exercising with a video, jumping rope, swimming and doing stationary exercises on specialized equipment such as a cross-country ski machine, elliptical machine, rowing machine, stairclimber/stepper, stationary bicycle (upright or recumbent) and treadmill. Although this book is geared toward at-home training – thereby emphasizing indoor activities – it would be inappropriate if outdoor activities were excluded from the discussion. Popular outdoor activities that can be used to stimulate aerobic fitness include bicycling, cross-country skiing, jogging/running, rowing and walking. Most of these aerobic options are recreational activities that you can perform – and enjoy – throughout your lifetime.

In addition, you can improve your aerobic fitness by playing sports such as soccer, basketball and tennis. Remember, though, that your level of intensity can vary a great deal during these activities due to their discontinuous nature. The way these activities are structured also influences your level of intensity: Playing full-court basketball is generally more demanding than half-court basketball; playing a singles match is generally more demanding than a doubles match.

To avoid boredom, it's important for you to change your activities from time to time. Fortunately, aerobic training permits a large amount of variety in terms of your activity selections.

Photo 4-3: You can use a variety of activities to increase your aerobic fitness.

Each aerobic activity has its advantages and disadvantages. For instance, swimming is desirable because it's a no-impact, non-weightbearing activity – the water supports your bodyweight which eliminates the impact forces on your bones, joints and connective tissues. On the other hand, swimming requires a fairly high degree of proficiency. If you have poor swimming skills, your heart rate may exceed your recommended training zone in a struggle just to keep yourself afloat. And if you aren't skilled at swimming, you'll also tire very quickly. Therefore, swimming isn't a good aerobic option for anyone who has poor swimming fundamentals. But swimming represents an excellent choice if your skills are adequate.

In addition, some aerobic activities aren't advisable if you're prone to certain injuries or likely to complicate an existing orthopedic condition. For example, jumping rope is a high-impact, weightbearing activity that has a greater risk of orthopedic stress and overuse injuries than a low-impact, non-weightbearing activity. Thus, jumping rope isn't recommended if you're larger than average – larger due to either fat or muscle tissue – because of the excessive stress that's placed on your ankles, knees and lower back. Likewise, a woman who jumps rope during pregnancy may endanger her fetus. Furthermore, someone who has chronic low-back pain would be more comfortable cycling in a recumbent position – which offers support for the lower back thereby decreasing the amount of stress on the lumbar spine – instead of in the traditional upright position. So, the best advice for you is to select suitable aerobic activities that are enjoyable, compatible with your skill levels and orthopedically safe.

If you're a weekend warrior who's preparing for a specific event – such as running or swimming – the best activities to do are the ones that you're going to perform in competition. If you want to become a better runner, you must primarily run; if you want to become a better swimmer, you must primarily swim. Similarly, a sport such as basketball requires a great deal of running. Logically, then, the best way for you to prepare for basketball is to run. This is not to say that your aerobic training should only involve running. But it should receive some priority in your training.

Otherwise, the best aerobic activities are the ones that you enjoy the most. As long as it's orthopedically appropriate, the type of activity that you choose to strengthen your aerobic system isn't as critical as the frequency, intensity and duration of the activity. Your aerobic system doesn't know if you pedaled on a recumbent cycle one day and ran on a treadmill the next. The only thing that really matters is whether or not you applied a meaningful workload to your aerobic system.

APPROPRIATE AEROBIC TRAINING

In a nutshell, you should perform your aerobic training at a frequency, intensity and time that's developmentally appropriate and orthopedically safe while using suitable activities that require a sustained effort. If you're healthy, your specific training prescription is to perform aerobic activities 3 - 5 times per week [frequency] at 60 - 90% of your age-predicted maximum heart rate [intensity] for 20 - 60 minutes [time] using appropriate activities that require a prolonged effort [type]. Bear in mind that all of these guidelines must be included in your aerobic training in order for you to improve your aerobic fitness.

MEANINGFUL AEROBIC TRAINING

Over a period of time, you'll likely find that the same aerobic workout – which was originally difficult – can be performed with less effort. As you become more fit, your training heart rate will be lower for a given level of intensity. Because of this, you must increase your intensity as needed so that you're always training with an appropriate percentage of your maximum heart rate. In addition, your ability to maintain a higher training heart rate will become easier. As a result, it's important to understand that you need to make your aerobic training progressively more chal-

lenging to make further improvements in your aerobic fitness.

To ensure that you produce continued aerobic improvements, you can progressively overload your aerobic system by (1) completing the same distance at a faster pace (that is, in a shorter amount of time); (2) covering a greater distance at the same pace; or (3) gradually increasing both the distance and the pace. As an example, suppose that you cycled 4.0 miles in 20 minutes. In a future aerobic workout, you should try to either cycle 4.0 miles in less than 20 minutes, cycle more than 4.0 miles in 20 minutes or cycle slightly more than 4.0 miles in a little less than 20 minutes. Regardless of which tactic you employ, you made your aerobic system work harder than it was accustomed to working.

Consequently, it's vital that you keep accurate records of your aerobic performances. Maintaining records permits you to keep track of your progress thereby making your aerobic workouts more productive and more meaningful. During aerobic training, the key program components to monitor include the date of your workout, the duration of your workout, the distance that you completed and the level of your intensity – that is, your training heart rate. (Appendix C contains a sample workout card for aerobic training.)

PREDICTING OXYGEN INTAKE

Oxygen intake (or oxygen consumption) is a very reliable and widely accepted indicator of

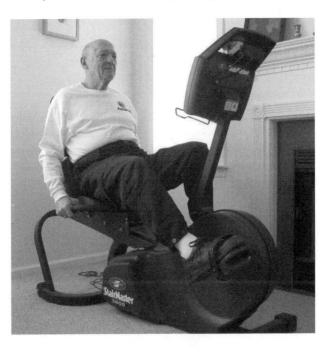

Photo 4-4: Someone who has chronic low-back pain would be more comfortable cycling in a recumbent position instead of in the traditional upright position.

TIME	VALUE	TIME	VALUE	TIME	VALUE	TIME	VALUE
8:00	63.84	10:00	51.77	12:00	43.73	14:00	37.98
8:05	63.22	10:05	51.37	12:05	43.45	14:05	37.77
8:10	62.61	10:10	50.98	12:10	43.17	14:10	37.57
8:15	62.01	10:15	50.59	12:15	42.90	14:15	37.37
8:20	61.42	10:20	50.21	12:20	42.64	14:20	37.18
8:25	60.85	10:25	49.84	12:25	42.38	14:25	36.98
8:30	60.29	10:30	49.47	12:30	42.12	14:30	36.79
8:35	59.74	10:35	49.11	12:35	41.86	14:35	36.60
8:40	59.20	10:40	48.75	12:40	41.61	14:40	36.41
8:45	58.67	10:45	48.40	12:45	41.36	14:45	36.23
8:50	58.15	10:50	48.06	12:50	41.11	14:50	36.04
8:55	57.63	10:55	47.72	12:55	40.87	14:55	35.86
9:00	57.13	11:00	47.38	13:00	40.63	15:00	35.68
9:05	56.64	11:05	47.05	13:05	40.39	15:05	35.50
9:10	56.16	11:10	46.73	13:10	40.16	15:10	35.33
9:15	55.68	11:15	46.41	13:15	39.93	15:15	35.15
9:20	55.21	11:20	46.09	13:20	39.70	15:20	34.98
9:25	54.76	11:25	45.78	13:25	39.48	15:25	34.81
9:30	54.31	11:30	45.47	13:30	39.26	15:30	34.64
9:35	53.87	11:35	45.17	13:35	39.04	15:35	34.48
9:40	53.43	11:40	44.87	13:40	38.82	15:40	34.31
9:45	53.01	11:45	44.58	13:45	38.61	15:45	34.15
9:50	52.59	11:50	44.29	13:50	38.39	15:50	33.99
9:55	52.18	11:55	44.01	13:55	38.19	15:55	33.83

TABLE 4.1: PREDICTED VALUES OF OXYGEN INTAKE (in ml/kg/min) BASED UPON THE TIME TO COMPLETE A 1.5-MILE RUN ON A LEVEL SURFACE

your aerobic fitness. Like virtually all of your other physiological characteristics, your aerobic potential is greatly influenced by your genetics. Your oxygen intake is also affected by your age, gender and body size.

One of the most simple and convenient tests that can be done to estimate your oxygen intake is the 1.5-Mile Running Test. The primary objective of this "field test" is to run 1.5 miles in the least amount of time. For the results to be as accurate as possible, you must run exactly 1.5 miles and it must be on a level (or horizontal) surface.

Because of this, running on an indoor or outdoor track is preferred. Generally, the results of the 1.5-Mile Running Test are an excellent predictor of your oxygen intake. But it's important to realize that this particular test of aerobic fitness favors runners since it involves running.

Table 4.1 lists predicted values of oxygen intake based upon the time that you take to complete a 1.5-mile run on a level surface. Various running times are given in five-second intervals from 8:00 - 15:55. These values are a relative measure of how much oxygen you consumed in

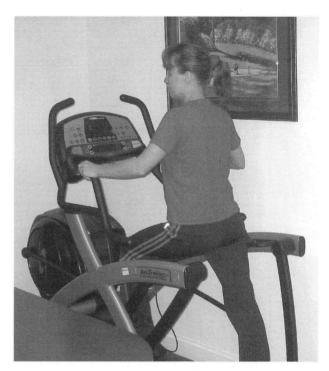

milliliters per kilogram of your bodyweight per minute (or ml/kg/min).

Oxygen Consumption: Relative

Let's suppose that a 30-year-old man weighs 198 pounds and can run 1.5 miles in 12:30. Note in Table 4.1 that his oxygen intake for this particular running time is 42.12 ml/kg/min – or simply 42.12. In other words, he consumed about 42.12 milliliters of oxygen for every kilogram that he weighed during each minute of his 1.5-mile run.

Table 4.2 shows norms for oxygen intake in relative terms for men and women of various ages. Referring to this table, note that this value [42.12 ml/kg/min] would be considered to be an "average" level of aerobic fitness for men who are in their 30s. (Elite male endurance athletes – such as cross-country runners, skiers and cyclists – have recorded values as high as the low 80s.)

Oxygen Consumption: Absolute

Oxygen intake can also be expressed in absolute terms in liters per minute (L/min). To determine your oxygen intake in L/min, you must first convert your bodyweight to kilograms (kg). To do this, divide your bodyweight in pounds (lb) by 2.2. Using the earlier example of the 30-year-old man, his 198-pound bodyweight is equal to 90 kg [198 lb ÷ 2.2 kg/lb = 90 kg]. Next, multiply his bodyweight (in kilograms) by his oxygen intake (in ml/kg/min) and divide by 1,000 (to convert from milliliters to liters). Staying with the same example as before yields a value of 3,790.8 ml/min [90 kg x 42.12 ml/kg/min = 3,790.8 ml/min]. To divide by 1,000, simply move the decimal point three places to the left. This means that a 198-pound individual who ran 1.5 miles in 12:30 would consume about 3.79 liters of oxygen during every minute of his run.

Table 4.3 shows norms for oxygen intake in absolute terms for men and women of various ages. Referring to this table, note that this value [3.79 L/min] would be considered to be a "high" level of fitness for men who are in their 30s. Recall that when his bodyweight wasn't considered, his level of aerobic fitness was considered "aver-

age." As such, oxygen intake in absolute terms gives a truer indication of aerobic fitness. (Values of more than 5.0 - 6.0 L/min are fairly common in highly fit individuals.)

It's important to note that the purpose of assessing your aerobic fitness isn't to compare your performance to that of another. It's unfair to make comparisons between individuals because everyone has a different genetic potential for achieving aerobic fitness. Assessments of fitness are more meaningful and fair when your performance is compared to your last performance – not to the performance of others.

ESTIMATING CALORIC EXPENDITURE

Essentially, a calorie is a unit of energy. In scientific terms, a calorie is defined as "the amount of heat required to raise the temperature of one gram of water by one degree Celsius." In practical terms, a calorie is a measure of your energy intake (eating) and your energy expenditure (exercising).

For all practical purposes, you use about 5.0 calories for every liter of oxygen that you consume. To determine your rate of caloric expenditure, simply take your oxygen intake in L/min and multiply it by 5.0 calories per liter (cal/L). Recall the earlier example of the 198-pound man whose oxygen intake was 3.79 L/min. In this case, his rate of caloric expenditure would be almost

MEN	LEVEL OF AEROBIC FITNESS				
Age	Low	Fair	Average	Good	High
20 - 29	<38	39 - 43	44 - 51	52 - 56	57+
30 - 39	<34	35 - 39	40 - 47	48 - 51	52+
40 - 49	<30	31 - 35	36 - 43	44 - 47	48+
50 - 59	<25	26 - 31	32 - 39	40 - 43	44+
60 - 69	<21	22 - 26	27 - 35	36 - 39	40+
WOMEN	**LEVEL OF AEROBIC FITNESS**				
Age	Low	Fair	Average	Good	High
20 - 29	<28	29 - 34	35 - 43	44 - 48	49+
30 - 39	<27	28 - 33	34 - 41	42 - 47	48+
40 - 49	<25	26 - 31	32 - 40	41 - 45	46+
50 - 65	<21	22 - 28	29 - 36	37 - 41	42+

TABLE 4.2: NORMS FOR OXYGEN INTAKE IN RELATIVE TERMS (in ml/kg/min) FOR MEN AND WOMEN

MEN	LEVEL OF AEROBIC FITNESS				
Age	Low	Fair	Average	Good	High
20 - 29	<2.79	2.80 - 3.09	3.10 - 3.69	3.70 - 3.99	4.00+
30 - 39	<2.49	2.50 - 2.79	2.80 - 3.39	3.40 - 3.69	3.70+
40 - 49	<2.19	2.20 - 2.49	2.50 - 3.09	3.10 - 3.39	3.40+
50 - 59	<1.89	1.90 - 2.19	2.20 - 2.79	2.80 - 3.09	3.10+
60 - 69	<1.59	1.60 - 1.89	1.90 - 2.49	2.50 - 2.79	2.80+
WOMEN	**LEVEL OF AEROBIC FITNESS**				
Age	Low	Fair	Average	Good	High
20 - 29	<1.69	1.70 - 1.99	2.00 - 2.49	2.50 - 2.79	2.80+
30 - 39	<1.59	1.60 - 1.89	1.90 - 2.39	2.40 - 2.69	2.70+
40 - 49	<1.49	1.50 - 1.79	1.80 - 2.29	2.30 - 2.59	2.60+
50 - 65	<1.29	1.30 - 1.59	1.60 - 2.09	2.10 - 2.39	2.40+

TABLE 4.3: NORMS FOR OXYGEN INTAKE IN ABSOLUTE TERMS (in L/min) FOR MEN AND WOMEN

19.0 calories per minute [3.79 L/min x 5.0 cal/L = 18.95 cal/min].

To determine the total number of calories that he used during his 1.5-mile run, multiply his rate of caloric expenditure (in cal/min) by his running time. In this case, multiplying 18.95 cal/min by 12.5 minutes (12:30 in decimal form) indicates that he used about 237.0 calories during his run [18.95 cal/min x 12.5 min = 236.88 cal].

5

INCREASING YOUR MUSCULAR STRENGTH

There are many benefits to strength training. First of all, increasing your muscular strength will improve your capacity to perform everyday tasks more easily. Strength training will also increase your muscle mass and decrease your body fat which will improve your body composition and physical appearance. In addition, strength training will increase your bone mineral density, thereby combating the destructive effects of osteoporosis. There are psychological benefits as well including increased mental alertness, self-confidence and self-esteem.

Most fitness authorities agree that strength training can be extremely beneficial. Many, however, disagree over which approach is best for increasing muscular strength (and size). The different approaches – and the abundant amount of conflicting information – often leave people quite confused.

In our society, time has truly become a precious commodity. Clearly, most people simply don't have an abundance of free time. After all, isn't that one of the main reasons why you've chosen to train in your home? Because of this limitation, you should seek and implement a strength-training program that produces the maximum possible results in the minimum amount of time. Therefore, efficiency should be a major consideration in developing your strength-training program. Another important consideration, of course, is safety. It makes little sense to do a program if it has a high potential for injury.

Interestingly, science has been unable to determine that one strength-training method is superior to another. Research has only shown that a variety of methods can increase muscular strength. One researcher, for example, found that similar increases in muscular strength were produced by nine different training routines consisting of various combinations of sets and repetitions. Increases in muscular strength can also be produced by a variety of equipment. Many studies have shown that groups using free weights and groups using machines produced similar improvements in muscular strength.

BLUEPRINT FOR STRENGTH

Since just about any type of program or equipment can produce favorable results, you must decide what's most practical for you based upon safety and time considerations. You can construct an efficient and effective strength-training program to utilize in your home gym – using virtually any type of equipment – by applying the information in the following blueprint for strength.

The Level of Intensity

The most important factor that determines your results from strength training is your genetic (or inherited) characteristics (which include the insertion points of your tendons, your predominant muscle-fiber type and so on). Unfortunately, you cannot control the genetic cards that you were dealt. The most important factor that you *can* control is your level of intensity. (With respect to strength training, "intensity" shouldn't be confused with "a percentage of a maximum weight." Rather, "intensity" is another word for "effort.")

A high level of intensity is necessary for maximizing your response to strength training. This level of effort is characterized by performing each set to the point of muscular fatigue or "failure." In simple terms, this means that you've exhausted your muscles to the extent that you literally cannot raise the weight for any additional repetitions.

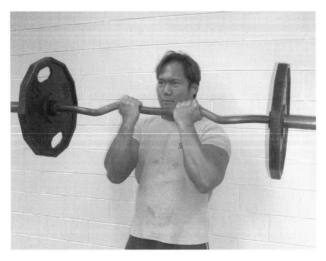

If you fail to reach a desirable level of intensity – or muscular fatigue – your increases in muscular strength (and size) will be less than optimal. Evidence for this "threshold" is found in the Overload Principle. This principle states that in order to increase muscular size and strength, a muscle must be stressed – or "overloaded" – with a workload that's beyond its present capacity.

Stated otherwise, you must produce a minimum level of muscular fatigue in order to provide a stimulus for adaptation. Your effort must be great enough to surpass this threshold so that a sufficient amount of muscular fatigue is created to trigger an adaptation. Given proper nourishment and an adequate amount of recovery between workouts, your muscles will adapt to these demands by increasing in strength (and size). The extent to which this "compensatory adaptation" occurs then becomes a function of your inherited characteristics.

So if you produce too little muscular fatigue, then you may not have stimulated any adaptation. But if you produce too much muscular fatigue, then you may not have permitted any adaptation; it may even cause a loss in muscular strength (and size). Therefore, your level of intensity should be high . . . but it should also be appropriate. To better appreciate the concept of using an appropriate level of intensity, consider this analogy: If you used a shovel on a regular basis for a short period of time, you'd form calluses on your palms. Basically, the calluses are a compensatory (and protective) adaptation to frictional heat. If you shoveled for a long enough period of time, however, you'd develop blisters instead. Here, the excessive demands have surpassed the adaptive ability of your epithelial tissue because the stress was too much. In brief, you should train with a high level of intensity without overdoing it.

How do you know if the demands on your muscles are too little or too much? You should monitor your performance in terms of the resistance that you use and the repetitions that you do. If you continue to make progress in your performance, then the demands are appropriate.

That being said, you must also use your judgment in deciding what level of intensity is suitable for you. "Intensity" is a relative term that depends upon your current level of fitness. Exercise of low intensity for an active individual may be of high intensity for an inactive individual. So if you haven't been training on a regular basis or aren't in the best of shape, then you should adjust your effort accordingly. Remember, you can control your level of intensity when you train: Your efforts can be as easy or as difficult as you desire.

Progressive Overload

It's not uncommon to hear of someone who performs the same number of repetitions with the same amount of resistance over and over again, workout after workout. Suppose that today you did a set of the bicep curl for 10 repetitions with 50 pounds and a month later you're still doing 10 repetitions with 50 pounds. Did you increase your strength? Probably not. On the other hand, what if you were able to do 11 repetitions with 60 pounds a month later? In this case, you were able to perform 10% more repetitions with 20% more resistance.

You must overload your muscles with progressively greater demands. For this reason, your muscles must experience a workload that's increased steadily and systematically throughout the course of your strength-training program. This is often referred to as "progressive overload."

In order to overload your muscles, every time you train you must attempt to increase the resistance that you use or the repetitions that you perform in comparison to your previous workout. Stated otherwise, you must impose demands upon your muscles that they haven't previously experienced by using more resistance or performing more repetitions. Exposing your muscles to progressively greater demands stimulates compensatory adaptation in response to the unaccustomed workload. Specifically, your muscles adapt to such demands by increasing in strength (and size).

In a nutshell, progressive overload would be accomplished in this manner: If you reach muscular fatigue within your prescribed repetition range – say that your range is 15 - 20 and you did 18 repetitions – you should repeat the resistance for your next workout and try to improve upon the number of repetitions that you did; if you attain or surpass the maximum number of prescribed repetitions in an exercise – say that your range is 10 - 15 and you did 15 repetitions – you should increase the resistance for your next workout.

You should increase the resistance in an amount with which you're comfortable . . . but the resistance that you use must always be challenging. Your muscles will respond better if the progressions in resistance are about 5% or less (depending upon the degree to which the exercise was challenging).

Number of Sets

For many years, most people have done multiple-set training simply because that's what they've read or been told to do. The roots of this advice can be traced back to the time when virtually every authority in strength training came from the ranks of the professional strongmen, competitive weightlifters and, to a lesser degree, bodybuilders. In the early 1970s, the notion was advanced that people could improve their strength (and size) with far fewer sets – and, thus, less volume of training – than had been traditionally thought.

Know this: Science has been unable to determine how many sets of each exercise are necessary to produce optimal increases in muscular

Photo 5-2: The overwhelming majority of scientific evidence indicates that single-set training is at least as effective as multiple-set training.

strength (and size). But the overwhelming majority of scientific evidence indicates that single-set training is at least as effective as multiple-set training. An exhaustive literature review in 1998 by Drs. Ralph Carpinelli and Robert Otto of Adelphi University (New York) and later reviews by Dr. Carpinelli examined all studies that compared different numbers of sets (dating back to 1956). Collectively, their research found 5 studies that showed multiple-set training was superior to single-set training *and 57 that did not.* And two of the studies that concluded multiple-set training was superior to single-set training involved only one exercise.

So, the basis for performing single-set training – or a relatively low number of sets – has powerful and compelling support in the scientific literature. But is single-set training actually done in the "real world"? More importantly, can experienced or "trained" individuals obtain the same results from single-set training as they can from multiple-set training? The answer to both questions is "yes." The fact of the matter is that single-set training has been popular since the early 1970s. And to quote Drs. Carpinelli and Otto: "There is no evidence to suggest that the response to single or multiple sets in trained athletes would differ from that in untrained individuals." Indeed, numerous authorities advocate single-set training including the strength coaches for many collegiate and professional teams. Dan Riley – a veteran strength coach with more than 20 years of experience in the National Football League and another 8 at the collegiate level (Penn

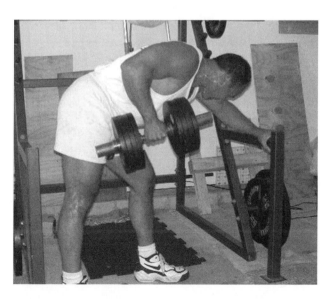

State and Army) – offers this advice to his players: "Your goal must be to perform as few sets as possible while stimulating maximum gains. If performed properly, only one set is needed to generate maximum gains. In our standard routines, one set of each exercise is performed."

Recall that in order for your muscles to increase in strength (and size), they must experience an adequate level of fatigue. It's just that simple. It really doesn't matter whether your muscles are fatigued in one set or several sets – as long as you produce a sufficient level of muscular fatigue.

If doing one set of an exercise produces virtually the same results as several sets, then single-set training represents a more efficient means of strength training. After all, why perform several sets when you can obtain similar results from one set in a fraction of the time? There's one caveat, however: If a single set of an exercise is to be productive, the set must be done with an appropriate level of intensity – that is, to the point of muscular fatigue. Your muscles should be thoroughly exhausted at the end of each exercise.

This is not to say that multiple-set training cannot be done. If performed properly, multiple-set training can certainly be effective in overloading your muscles. If you have a preference for multiple-set training, you should be aware of several things. First of all, simply doing multiple sets doesn't guarantee that you've overloaded your muscles. If the weights you use aren't demanding enough, then you will not produce sufficient muscular fatigue and your workout will not be as effective as possible. Remember, a large amount of low-intensity work doesn't necessarily produce an overload. So if you'd rather do multiple sets, make sure that you're challenging your muscles with a progressive overload. In addition, keep in mind that performing too many sets (or too many exercises) can create a situation in which the demands on your muscles have surpassed your ability to recover. If this happens, your muscle tissue will be broken down in such an extreme manner that your body is unable to adapt to the demands. Also, doing too many sets (or too many exercises) can significantly increase your risk of incurring an overuse injury such as tendinitis and bursitis. And multiple-set training is relatively inefficient in terms of time so it's un-

desirable for time-conscious individuals. The point is this: Keep your sets to the minimum amount that's needed to produce an adequate level of muscular fatigue.

You should emphasize the *quality* of work that you do rather than the *quantity* of work. Don't perform meaningless sets – make every set count.

Number of Repetitions

Determining an appropriate repetition range depends upon a number of factors and, even then, has some degree of variability. Understand first that strength training isn't an aerobic activity that's characterized by long-term, low-intensity efforts. Rather, it's an anaerobic activity that's characterized by short-term, high-intensity efforts. Therefore, the duration of a series of repetitions – that is, a set – should be in the anaerobic domain. Efforts that last from a split second to several minutes are considered to be anaerobic (assuming, of course, that the level of effort is great enough to justify an anaerobic response). Since intense efforts at the lower end of this time frame carry a higher risk of injury and those at the upper end have a greater reliance on the aerobic pathways, narrowing the window of time to roughly 40 - 120 seconds represents a safe and effective range for strength training with higher durations assigned to larger muscles and lower durations to smaller ones. (Larger muscles – such as those in your hips and legs – should be trained for a slightly longer duration because of their greater size and work capacity.) Thus, time frames might be 90 - 120 seconds for a hip exercise, 60 - 90 seconds for a leg exercise and 40 - 70 seconds for a torso exercise.

Be that as it may, doing sets for a specified amount of time can be tricky and tedious. But you can use the aforementioned time frames to formulate repetition ranges. Suppose that you prefer to use a speed of movement that's six seconds per repetition. Dividing six seconds into the time frames that have been noted yields the following repetition ranges: 15 - 20 for your hips, 10 - 15 for your legs and about 6 - 12 for your torso. (A minimum of 8 repetitions is recommended for torso exercises that have a short range of motion). Remember, these ranges are based upon six-second repetitions. Different repetition speeds require different repetition ranges. Suppose that you prefer to use a speed of movement that's 10 seconds per repetition. Dividing 10 seconds into the time frames that were mentioned earlier results in the following repetition ranges: 9 - 12 for your hips, 6 - 9 for your legs and about 4 - 7 for your torso. (You're encouraged to experiment with different repetition speeds and vary them based upon your personal preferences.)

A final point: It's safer for certain populations to perform more repetitions than have been suggested in order to reduce orthopedic stress. Slightly higher repetition ranges are recommended for younger teenagers and older adults (particularly those with hypertension) along with anyone doing rehabilitative training. For example, repetition ranges might be 20 - 25 for exercises involving the hips, 15 - 20 for the legs and 10 - 15 for the torso. These higher repetition ranges necessitate using somewhat lighter weights which reduces the orthopedic stress placed upon the bones and connective tissues.

Proper Technique

The technique that you use to perform your repetitions is critical to the success of your strength-training program. Clearly, *how well* you lift a weight is more important than *how much* weight you lift.

A repetition has four checkpoints: the positive (or raising) phase, the mid-range position, the negative (or lowering) phase and the range of motion.

Checkpoint #1

A repetition starts with the raising of the weight. You should raise the weight in a deliberate, controlled manner without any explosive or jerking movements.

Raising a weight in a rapid, explosive fashion isn't recommended for two main reasons. First of all, high-speed repetitions that are performed in a ballistic manner are actually less productive than low-speed repetitions that are performed in a controlled manner. Here's why: When weights are lifted explosively, the muscles pro-

duce tension during the initial part of the movement . . . but not for the last part. In simple terms, the weight is practically moving by itself. In effect, the load on the muscles is decreased – or eliminated – and so are the potential gains in muscular strength (and size).

As an example, imagine that you raised the weight so quickly on a leg-extension machine that the pad left your lower legs partway through the repetition. Think about it: The pad is attached to the movement arm of the machine that, in turn, is connected to the resistance by some means (such as a chain, cable or belt). If the pad is no longer in contact with your lower legs, there's no load on your muscles. If there's no load on your muscles, there's no stimulus – or reason – for them to adapt. Sure, you will obtain some benefit when your muscles were loaded during the first part of the repetition (when the pad was against your shins). However, you will not obtain any benefit when your muscles were *unloaded* during the last part of the repetition (when the pad left your shins).

Secondly – and more importantly – high-speed repetitions also carry a greater risk of injury than low-speed repetitions. Raising a weight too fast increases the shearing forces encountered by a given joint; the faster a weight is raised, the higher these forces are amplified. In one study, a subject who squatted with 80% of his four-rep-

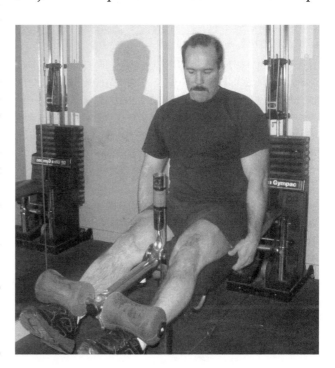

Photo 5-3: The technique that you use to perform your repetitions is critical to the success of your strength-training program.

etition maximum incurred a 225-pound peak shearing force during a repetition that took 4.5 seconds to complete and a 270-pound peak shearing force during a repetition that took 2.1 seconds to complete. This is clear evidence that a slower speed of movement reduces the shearing forces on joints. When the forces exceed the structural limits of a joint, an injury occurs to the muscles, connective tissues or bones. To ensure that your repetitions are safe and productive, it should take at least 1 - 2 seconds to raise the weight to the mid-range position.

Checkpoint #2

After raising the weight, you should pause briefly in the position of full muscular contraction or the mid-range position. Where's the mid-range position of a repetition? These two examples should help make it clear: When performing a leg extension, the mid-range position is where your legs are completely extended (or as straight as possible); when performing a bicep curl, the mid-range position is where your arms are completely flexed (or as bent as possible).

Most people are very weak in the mid-range position of a repetition because they rarely, if ever, emphasize it. Pausing momentarily in the mid-range position allows you to focus your attention on your muscles when they're fully contracted. Furthermore, a brief pause in the mid-range position permits a smooth transition between the raising and lowering of the weight.

Checkpoint #3

A repetition ends with the lowering of the weight. The importance of emphasizing the negative phase of a repetition cannot be overstated. Numerous studies have reported that repetitions involving both raising and lowering a weight produce greater increases in strength (and size) than those involving just raising.

Remember, the same muscles that you use to raise a weight are also used to lower it. In a bicep curl, for example, your biceps are used in raising and lowering the weight. The only difference is that when you raise the weight, your biceps are shortening against the load and when you lower the weight, your biceps are lengthening against the load. So by emphasizing the lowering of the weight, each repetition becomes more productive. Because a "loaded" muscle length-

ens as you lower a weight, emphasizing the negative phase of a repetition also ensures that the exercised muscle is being stretched properly and safely.

In any given exercise, you can lower more weight than you can raise. It stands to reason, then, that the lowering of the weight should take more time to complete than the raising of the weight. To ensure that your repetitions are safe and productive, it should take at least 3 - 4 seconds to lower the weight back to the starting position.

Effectively, it should take at least 4 - 6 seconds to perform a productive repetition. One study demonstrated a 50% increase in upper-body strength and a 33% increase in lower-body strength in a group that performed each repetition by raising the weight in two seconds and lowering it in four seconds. Furthermore, two additional studies reported average increases in muscular strength of 55% in 17 subjects and 58.2% in 31 subjects. In both of these studies, the subjects used the same six-second guideline to raise and lower the weight.

Checkpoint #4

A repetition should be done throughout the greatest possible range of motion that safety allows – from a full stretch to a full muscular contraction and back to a full stretch. Doing your repetitions throughout a full range of motion will allow you to maintain (or perhaps increase) your flexibility. Moreover, it ensures that you're stimulating your entire muscle – not just a portion of it – thereby making the repetitions more productive. Clearly, doing full-range repetitions is a requirement for obtaining full-range effects.

Duration of the Workout

When it comes to strength training, more isn't necessarily better. Be aware that an inverse relationship exists between time and intensity: As the time of an activity increases, the level of intensity decreases. Stated otherwise, you cannot possibly train with a high level of intensity for a long period of time. If you lengthen the duration of your workout – by increasing either the number of exercises or sets that you normally perform – you must reduce your level of intensity. And, of course, using a lower level of intensity isn't desirable.

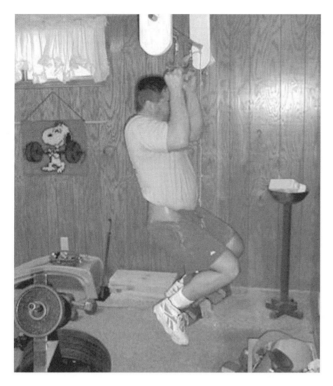

Photo 5-4: You can make your workouts more efficient – and more intense – by taking as little recovery as possible between exercises/sets.

It's important to note that carbohydrates are your preferred fuel during intense activity. Carbohydrates circulate in your bloodstream as glucose and are stored in your liver and muscles as glycogen. Most people exhaust their carbohydrate stores after about one hour of intense activity. For this reason, your strength training should be completed in approximately one hour or less. (Note that this one-hour window of time will dictate the number of exercises and sets that you can perform in your workout.)

The exact duration of your workout depends upon several factors such as the transition time to prepare for each exercise/set (such as changing plates, moving pins and so on) and the recovery time between each exercise/set. Generally speaking, however, you should be able to complete your workout in no more than about one hour.

You can make your workouts more efficient – and more intense – by taking as little recovery as possible between exercises/sets. The length of your recovery interval depends upon your current level of fitness. Initially, you may require several minutes of recovery between exercises/sets to "catch your breath" or feel that you can produce a maximal level of effort. With improved fitness, your pace can be quickened to the point where you're moving as quickly as possible be-

tween exercises/sets. (The speed with which you do your repetitions shouldn't be quickened – just the pace between exercises/sets.)

Volume of Exercises

Most people can perform a comprehensive, total-body workout using 14 exercises or less. The focal point for most of these exercises should be your major muscle groups (that is, your hips, legs and torso). Include one exercise for your hips, hamstrings, quadriceps, calves/dorsi flexors, biceps, triceps, abdominals and lower back. Because your shoulder joint allows movement at many different angles, you should perform two exercises for your chest, upper back (your "lats") and shoulders. You can choose any exercises that you prefer in order to address those body parts.

For some "weekend warriors," a thorough workout may require slightly more than 14 exercises. For instance, if you participate in a sport or activity that requires grip strength – such as softball or golf – your workout should include one exercise for your forearms. (A summary of the recommended volume of exercises and repetition ranges is given in Figure 5.1.)

Once again, more isn't necessarily better when it comes to strength training. Performing too many exercises can produce too much stress which will impede progress. A total-body workout that contains 20 exercises could be devastating for someone who has a low level of tolerance for strength training. And the more exercises that you perform, the more difficult it will be for you to maintain a desirable level of intensity.

This is not to say that you cannot do an extra exercise or two in order to emphasize a particular body part. As long as you continue to make improvements in your strength, you aren't performing too many exercises. So if your workout consists of 20 exercises and you're making progress, then you aren't overtraining. But if you start to level off or "plateau" in one or more exercises, it's probably because you're overtraining – the volume of your training has exceeded your ability to recover.

BODY PART	EXERCISES	REPETITION RANGE
Hips	1	15 - 20
Hamstrings	1	10 - 15
Quadriceps	1	10 - 15
Calves or Dorsi Flexors	1	10 - 15
Chest	2	6 - 12
Upper Back (or "lats")	2	6 - 12
Shoulders	2	6 - 12 or 8 - 12
Biceps	1	6 - 12
Triceps	1	6 - 12
Forearms (optional)	1	8 - 12
Abdominals	1	8 - 12 or 10 - 12
Lower Back	1	10 - 15

FIGURE 5.1: SUMMARY OF THE RECOMMENDED VOLUME OF EXERCISES AND REPETITION RANGES

Sequence of Exercises

The order in which you perform your exercises is essential in producing optimal improvements in your muscular strength (and size). As a rule of thumb, the idea is to train your most important muscles as early as possible in your workout. It stands to reason that you should address those muscles while you're fresh, both mentally as well as physically. In effect, your workout should begin with exercises that influence your largest muscles and proceed to those that involve your smallest ones.

In a total-body workout, the best order of exercise would usually look like this: hips, upper legs (hamstrings and quadriceps), lower legs (calves or dorsi flexors), torso (chest, upper back and shoulders), upper arms (biceps and triceps), abdominals and finally your lower back. If performed, exercises for the lower arms (the forearms) would be done after those for the upper arms.

If you prefer to do a "split routine" – in which you "split" your body parts into several workouts instead of one total-body workout – the aforementioned order of exercise would still apply. In a workout that only targeted the chest, shoulders and triceps, for example, you should still address those body parts from largest to smallest.

Frequency of Training

Intense strength training places great demands upon your muscles. In order to adapt to those demands, your muscles must receive an adequate amount of recovery between your workouts.

Adaptation to the demands occurs during the recovery process. Believe it or not, your muscles don't get stronger during your workout . . . your muscles get stronger *after* your workout. If the demands are of sufficient magnitude, a muscle is literally torn. Although these tears are quite small – microscopic, in fact – the recovery process is essential in that it allows the damaged muscle enough time to repair itself. Think of this as allowing a wound to heal. If you had a scab and picked at it every day, you'd delay the healing process. But if you left it alone, you'd permit the damaged tissue time to heal. So in a sense, the recovery following a workout is a process in which damaged tissue – in this case, muscle tissue – is healed.

There are individual variations in recovery ability – everyone has different levels of tolerance for exercise. However, a period of about 48 - 72 hours is usually necessary for muscle tissue to recover sufficiently from an intense strength-training workout.

Keep in mind, too, that intense training relies heavily upon carbohydrates as the primary source of energy. Adequate recovery is required to return the carbohydrate (or glycogen) stores to their pre-training levels. It appears as if about 48 hours are needed for this to be accomplished. As a result, it's suggested that you perform strength training 2 - 3 times per week on non-consecutive days such as on Monday, Wednesday and Friday. (Note that this assumes total-body workouts.)

Can you achieve significant improvements in strength by doing just two weekly workouts? Absolutely. In a study that involved 117 subjects, a group that trained two times per week experienced approximately 80% of the gains in strength of the group that trained three times per week.

An appropriate frequency (and volume) of strength training can be likened to doses of medication. In order for medicine to improve a condition, it must be taken at specific intervals and in certain amounts. Taking medicine at a greater frequency or in a larger quantity beyond what's needed can have harmful effects. Similarly, an "overdose" of strength training – in which workouts are done too often or have too much volume – can also be detrimental. Performing any more than three "doses" of total-body workouts per week will gradually become counterproductive.

How do you know if your muscles have had an adequate amount of recovery? You should see a gradual improvement in the amount of resistance and/or number of repetitions that you're able to do over the course of several weeks. If not, then you're probably not getting enough recovery between your workouts (which, again, could be the result of performing too many sets or too many exercises). Remember, strength training will be effective if it provides an *overload* not an *overdose*.

Record Keeping

If your strength training is to be as productive as possible, it's absolutely critical to keep written records that are as accurate and detailed as possible. Records document the history of what you accomplished during each and every exercise of each and every strength session. Because of this, maintaining records is an extremely valuable tool to monitor your progress and make your workouts more meaningful. Records can also be used to identify exercises in which you've reached a plateau. In the unfortunate event of an injury, you can also gauge the effectiveness of the rehabilitative process if you have a record of your pre-injury levels of strength.

A workout card can have an infinite number of appearances and need not be elaborate. However, you should be able to record your bodyweight, the date of each workout, the resistance used for each exercise, the number of repetitions performed for each exercise and the order in which the exercises were completed. The recommended repetition ranges should also be given for each exercise.

An illustration of how to record data on a workout card is shown in Figure 5.2. (Appendices D and E contain workout cards for single-set training and multiple-set training, respectively.)

The bottom line: Don't underestimate the importance of using a workout card in making your strength training more productive and more meaningful.

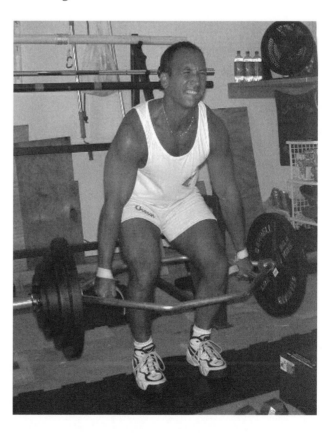

Photo 5-5: Your workout should begin with exercises that influence your largest muscles and proceed to those that involve your smallest ones.

NAME: I.M.Fitt		DATE	Mon 4/4	Wed 4/6	Fri 4/8	Mon 4/11	Wed 4/13
		BW	180	180	179	179	
	EXERCISE	REPS	wt / reps	wt / reps	wt / reps	wt / reps	wt / reps
HIPS (1)	Squat (ball)	15-20	BW / 18	BW / 20	BW+5 / 19		
	Deadlift	15-20				95 / 20	97.5 /
UPPER LEGS (2)	Prone Leg Curl	10-15	50 / 15	52.5 / 14	52.5 / 14	52.5 / 15	55 /
	Leg Extension	10-15	65 / 10	65 / 11	65 / 12	65 / 12	65 /
LOWER LEGS (1)	Seated Calf Raise	10-15	20 / 17	22.5 / 16	25 / 15	27.5 / 14	
	Dorsi Flexion	10-15					20
CHEST (2)	Bench Press	6-12	105 / 8	105 / 9	105 / 10	105 / 10	105 /
	Bent-Arm Fly	6-12	25 / 8	25 / 9	25 / 9	25 / 10	25 /

FIGURE 5.2: RECORDING WORKOUT DATA (SINGLE-SET TRAINING)

6

THE HIPS

Because such a large amount of muscle mass is located below your waist, it's generally the most important region in the body. Therefore, a comprehensive strength-training workout must address the muscles of the lower body – especially the hips.

MUSCLES OF THE HIPS

Your hip region is made up of three main muscle groups: the gluteals, adductors and iliopsoas.

Gluteals

Your gluteals (or "glutes") are located on the back of your hips. They're composed of three primary muscles: the gluteus maximus, gluteus medius and gluteus minimus. The largest and strongest muscle in your body is your gluteus maximus (which forms your buttocks or "butt"). The main function of this muscle is hip extension (driving your upper legs backward). Your gluteus medius and gluteus minimus cause hip abduction (spreading your legs apart). Your gluteal muscles are involved significantly in walking, running, jumping and stairclimbing.

Adductors

Your adductor group is composed of five muscles that are found throughout your inner thigh. The muscles of your inner thigh are used during hip adduction (bringing your legs together).

Iliopsoas

The "iliopsoas" is actually a collective term for the primary muscles on the front of your hips: the iliacus, psoas major and psoas minor. The main function of the iliopsoas is hip flexion (bringing your knees to your chest). Your iliopsoas has a major role in many activities such as lifting your knees when walking, running and stairclimbing. The iliopsoas is sometimes considered with the muscles of the abdomen. Because of this, exercises for the iliopsoas are also discussed with those of the abdominals (Chapter 14).

EXERCISES FOR THE HIPS

This chapter will describe and illustrate eight exercises that you can perform for your hip muscles. These exercises are the deadlift, squat (with a stability ball), leg press, lunge, lunge (with a stability ball), hip abduction (with a cable column), hip abduction (with an ankle/wrist weight) and hip adduction (with a cable column).

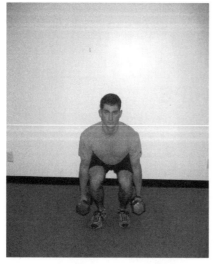
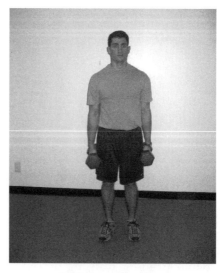

Start/Finish Position　　　　*Mid-Range Position*

DEADLIFT

Equipment Needed: dumbbells, barbell or trap bar

Muscles Influenced: gluteus maximus (buttocks), hamstrings, quadriceps and erector spinae (lower back)

Suggested Repetitions: 15 - 20

Start/Finish Position: Spread your feet slightly wider than shoulder-width apart. Reach down and grasp a dumbbell in each hand on the outside of your legs with a "parallel grip" (your palms facing each other). Lower your hips until your upper legs are almost parallel to the floor. Flatten your back and look up slightly. Place most of your bodyweight on your heels, not on the balls of your feet.

Performance Description: Stand upright by straightening your legs and torso. Pause briefly in this mid-range position (your hips, legs and torso extended) and then lower the weight under control to the start/finish position (your hips, legs and torso flexed) to ensure an adequate stretch.

Training Tips:

- Don't lift your hips too early as you perform this exercise. Raising your hips too soon causes you to do the exercise almost entirely with your lower back. Ideally, your hips, legs and lower back should work together. However, your hips and legs should do most of the work.

- You should exert force through your heels, not the balls of your feet.

- You shouldn't "lock" or "snap" your knees in the mid-range position of a repetition. This removes the load from the target muscles and may hyperextend your knees.

- Keep your arms straight, head up and back relatively flat as you perform this exercise.

- You can also perform this exercise with a barbell and trap bar. When doing this exercise with a barbell, you should use an "alternating grip" (your dominant palm forward and non-dominant palm backward). Otherwise, the exercise would be performed in the same fashion as described above.

- When using a barbell or trap bar, don't bounce the weight off the floor between repetitions.

- You can use wrist straps if you have difficulty in maintaining your grip on the dumbbells (or the bar).

- This exercise may be contraindicated if you have low-back pain, hyperextended elbows or an exceptionally long torso and/or legs.

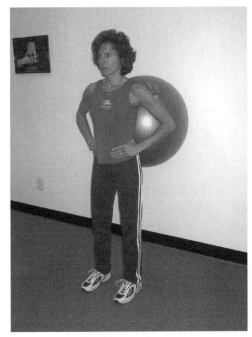
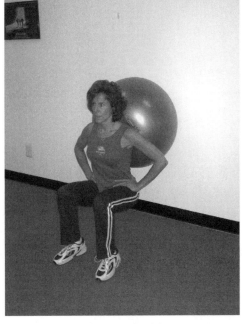

Start/Finish Position   *Mid-Range Position*

SQUAT (stability ball)

Equipment Needed: stability ball

Muscles Influenced: gluteus maximus, hamstrings and quadriceps

Suggested Repetitions: 15 - 20

Start/Finish Position: Stand up straight and place a stability ball behind your lower back against a smooth, unobstructed wall. Position your feet (as described below in the training tips) and spread them slightly wider than shoulder-width apart. Straighten your legs until they're almost fully extended (that is, without "locking" your knees). Interlock your fingers and place your palms against your mid-section (or place your hands on your hips). Place most of your bodyweight on your heels, not on the balls of your feet.

Performance Description: Lower yourself under control until the angle between your upper and lower legs is about 90 degrees. Without bouncing, return to the start/finish position (your legs almost fully extended).

Training Tips:

- Adjust the position of your feet so that your lower legs are perpendicular to the floor in the mid-range position.
- You shouldn't lower yourself to a depth in which the angle between your upper and lower legs is less than about 90 degrees.
- Don't bounce out of the mid-range position. Bouncing out of this position produces higher compressive loads and shear forces.
- You should exert force through your heels, not the balls of your feet.
- You shouldn't "lock" or "snap" your knees in the start/finish position of a repetition. This removes the load from the target muscles and may hyperextend your knees.
- This exercise can be performed with added resistance by holding a dumbbell in each hand on the outside of your legs.
- This exercise may be contraindicated if you have low-back pain.

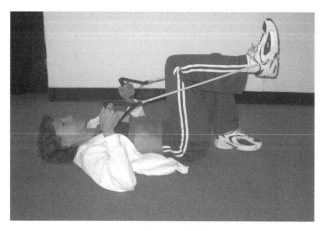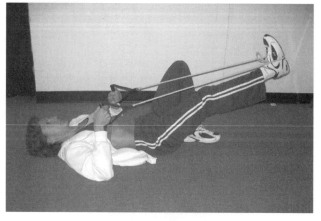

Start/Finish Position   Mid-Range Position

LEG PRESS

Equipment Needed: resistance band/cord

Muscles Influenced: gluteus maximus, hamstrings and quadriceps

Suggested Repetitions: 15 - 20

Start/Finish Position: Lie supine on the floor, grasp one end of a resistance band/cord in each hand and place the bottom of your right foot on the inside of it. Position your right upper leg so that it's roughly perpendicular to the floor. Adjust the position of your hands so that the band/cord is taut. Bend your left leg and place your left foot flat on the floor. Lay your head flat on the floor.

Performance Description: Push your right foot forward until your leg is almost fully extended (that is, without "locking" your knee). Pause briefly in this mid-range position (your hip and leg extended) and then return your leg under control to the start/finish position (your hip and leg flexed) to provide a proper stretch. After performing a set with your right leg, repeat the exercise for the other side of your body.

Training Tips:

• The middle of the band/cord should be positioned near the bottom of your foot just above the heel.

• You should exert force through your heel, not the ball of your foot.

• You shouldn't "lock" or "snap" your knee in the mid-range position of a repetition. This removes the load from the target muscles and may hyperextend your knee.

• If you can do 20 repetitions or more with strict form using a resistance band/cord, you can increase the workload on your muscles by using a band/cord of greater resistance, using multiple bands/cords or performing the exercise with a slower speed of movement.

• This exercise may be contraindicated if you have a hyperextended knee.

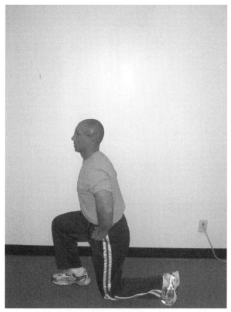
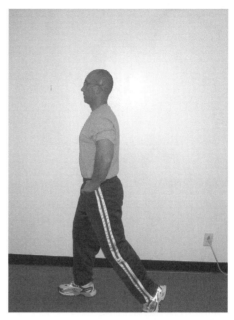

Start/Finish Position   *Mid-Range Position*

LUNGE

Equipment Needed: none

Muscles Influenced: gluteus maximus, hamstrings and quadriceps

Suggested Repetitions: 15 - 20

Start/Finish Position: Step forward with your right foot and point it straight ahead. Bend your left knee, drop your hips and position your right lower leg so that it's approximately perpendicular to the floor. Straighten your torso and place your hands on your hips.

Performance Description: Stand up by straightening your right leg while keeping it perpendicular to the floor. Pause briefly in this mid-range position (your right leg extended) and then lower yourself under control to the start/finish position (your right leg flexed) to ensure an adequate stretch. After performing a set with your right leg, repeat the exercise for the other side of your body.

Training Tips:

• Keep your lower leg of the forward foot perpendicular to the floor as you perform this exercise.

• This exercise can be performed with added resistance by holding a dumbbell in each hand on the outside of your legs.

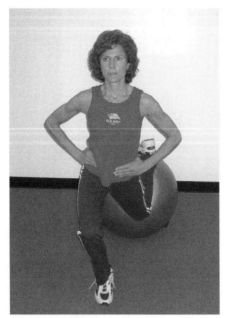
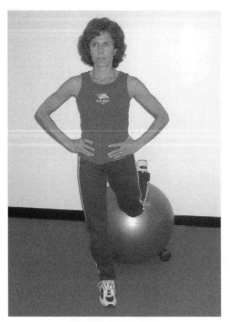

Start/Finish Position   *Mid-Range Position*

LUNGE (stability ball)

Equipment Needed: stability ball

Muscles Influenced: gluteus maximus, hamstrings and quadriceps

Suggested Repetitions: 15 - 20

Start/Finish Position: Step forward with your right foot and point it straight ahead. Place your left lower leg on a stability ball, drop your hips and position your right lower leg so that it's approximately perpendicular to the floor. Straighten your torso and place your hands on your hips.

Performance Description: Stand up by straightening your right leg while keeping it perpendicular to the floor. Pause briefly in this mid-range position (your right leg extended) and then lower yourself under control to the start/finish position (your right leg flexed) to ensure an adequate stretch. After performing a set with your right leg, repeat the exercise for the other side of your body.

Training Tips:

• You can place dumbbells alongside the ball to keep it in place.

• Keep your lower leg of the forward foot perpendicular to the floor as you perform this exercise.

• This exercise can be performed with added resistance by holding a dumbbell in each hand on the outside of your legs.

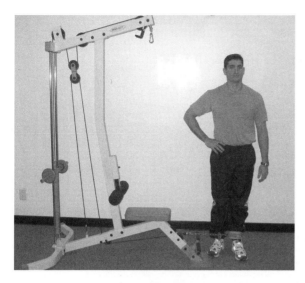 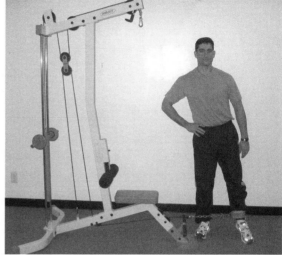

Start/Finish Position   *Mid-Range Position*

HIP ABDUCTION (cable column)

Equipment Needed: cable column and ankle/wrist strap

Muscle Influenced: gluteus medius

Suggested Repetitions: 10 - 15

Start/Finish Position: Adjust the position of the pulley so that it's near the bottom of the column and attach an ankle/wrist strap. Secure the ankle/wrist strap around your left ankle. Stand upright so that the right side of your body is facing the pulley. Slide your feet away from the machine so that the weight you intend to lift is separated slightly from the rest of the weight stack. Put your hands on your hips (or, if possible, put your right hand against the machine to stabilize your body) and place most of your weight on your right foot.

Performance Description: Without bending forward or to the right, raise your left leg as high as possible. Pause briefly in this mid-range position (your legs apart) and then lower the weight under control to the start/finish position (your legs together) to obtain a proper stretch. After performing a set with your left leg, repeat the exercise for the other side of your body.

Training Tips:

• Don't bend forward or laterally at the waist as you perform this exercise.

• Attempt to raise your leg as high as possible in the mid-range position of every repetition to ensure that you're obtaining a maximal contraction of the target muscles throughout the duration of the exercise.

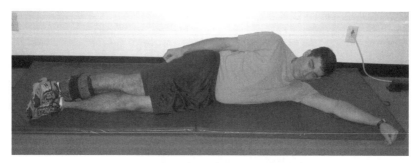

Start/Finish Position

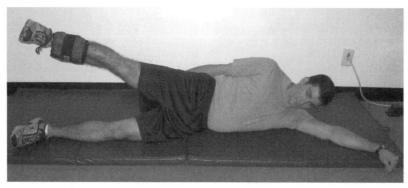

Mid-Range Position

HIP ABDUCTION (ankle/wrist weight)

Equipment Needed: ankle/wrist weight

Muscle Influenced: gluteus medius

Suggested Repetitions: 10 - 15

Start/Finish Position: Secure an ankle/wrist weight around your right ankle. Lie down on the floor on the left side of your body, straighten your legs and point your right toes toward your right knee. Extend your left arm across the floor.

Performance Description: Without bending forward, raise your right leg as high as possible. Pause briefly in this mid-range position (your legs apart) and then return the weight under control to the start/finish position (your legs together) to obtain a proper stretch. After performing a set with your right leg, repeat the exercise for the other side of your body (lying on the right side of your body).

Training Tips:

• Don't bend forward at the waist as you perform this exercise.

• Attempt to raise your leg as high as possible in the mid-range position of every repetition to ensure that you're obtaining a maximal contraction of the target muscles throughout the duration of the exercise.

• If you can do 15 repetitions or more with strict form using an ankle/wrist weight, you can increase the workload on your muscles by using a weight of greater resistance, using multiple weights or performing the exercise with a slower speed of movement.

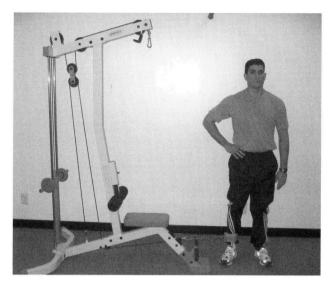
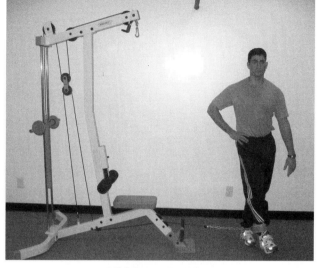

Start/Finish Position   *Mid-Range Position*

HIP ADDUCTION (cable column)

Equipment Needed: cable column and ankle/wrist strap

Muscles Influenced: hip adductors (inner thigh)

Suggested Repetitions: 10 - 15

Start/Finish Position: Adjust the position of the pulley so that it's near the bottom of the column and attach an ankle/wrist strap. Secure the ankle/wrist strap around your right ankle. Stand upright so that the right side of your body is facing the pulley. Slide your feet away from the machine so that the weight you intend to lift is separated slightly from the rest of the weight stack. Put your hands on your hips (or, if possible, put your right hand against the machine to stabilize your body), spread apart your feet and place most of your weight on your left foot.

Performance Description: Without bending forward or to the right, bring your right leg across the front of your left leg as far as possible. Pause briefly in this mid-range position (your legs crossed) and then return the weight under control to the start/finish position (your legs apart) to provide an adequate stretch. After performing a set with your right leg, repeat the exercise for the other side of your body.

Training Tips:

• Don't bend forward or laterally at the waist as you perform this exercise.

• Attempt to raise the weight as high as possible in the mid-range position of every repetition to ensure that you're obtaining a maximal contraction of the target muscles throughout the duration of the exercise.

• Don't slam the weights together between repetitions.

7

THE UPPER LEGS

A considerable amount of muscle mass is located in your upper legs. Because of this, these muscles shouldn't be neglected in a strength-training program.

MUSCLES OF THE UPPER LEGS

The two main muscle groups of your upper legs (or thighs) are the hamstrings and quadriceps.

Hamstrings

Your hamstrings (or "hams") are found on the back of your upper legs and actually include three muscles. Together, these muscles are involved in knee flexion (bringing your heels toward your buttocks) and hip extension (driving your upper legs backward). Your hamstrings are used extensively during virtually every running and jumping activity. One of the best reasons that you should strengthen your hamstrings is that they're quite susceptible to pulls and tears. Clearly, strong muscles on the back of your upper legs are necessary to counterbalance the powerful muscles on the front of your upper legs.

Quadriceps

Your quadriceps (or "quads") are the most important muscles on the front of your upper legs. As the name suggests, your quadriceps are made up of four muscles. The main function of your quadriceps is knee extension (straightening your legs). Your quadriceps are involved in all running, kicking and jumping skills.

EXERCISES FOR THE UPPER LEGS

This chapter will describe and illustrate four exercises that you can perform for the muscles of your upper legs. These exercises are the prone leg curl, seated leg curl, leg curl (with a stability ball) and leg extension.

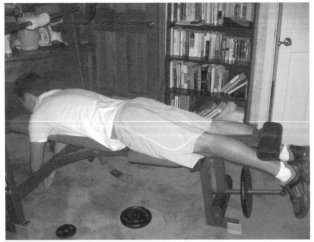
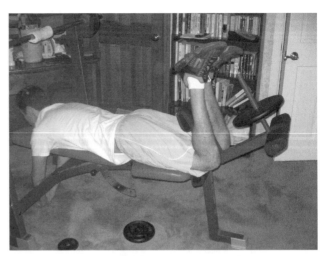

| Start/Finish Position | Mid-Range Position |

PRONE LEG CURL

Equipment Needed: resistance machine

Muscles Influenced: hamstrings

Suggested Repetitions: 10 - 15

Start/Finish Position: If possible, adjust the position of the leg pad (as described below in the training tips). Lie face down on the back pad and place your lower legs underneath the leg pad. Position the tops of your kneecaps so that they're just over the edge of the back pad, not on the pad. (By doing this, your knees will be approximately even with the axis of rotation of the machine.) If the machine has handles, lightly grasp them (or grasp the back pad).

Performance Description: Bring your heels as close to your hips as possible by pulling against the leg pad. Pause briefly in this mid-range position (your heels near your hips) and then lower the weight under control to the start/finish position (your legs fully extended) to ensure a sufficient stretch.

Training Tips:

- Adjust the position of the leg pad so that it's near the bottom part of your calves (just above your ankles) in the start/finish position. (Some machines have two leg pads rather than one.)

- Keep your torso against the back pad as you perform this exercise. You can raise your hips as you perform this exercise, however, since this actually increases your range of motion. Otherwise, movement should only occur around your knee joints.

- The angle between your upper and lower legs should be about 90 degrees or less in the mid-range position. This could be deceiving if the pad is humped or angled rather than parallel to the floor.

- Don't slam the weights together or bounce the movement arm against the machine between repetitions.

- You can do this exercise unilaterally (one limb at a time) if you have a leg or knee injury, a gross difference in the strength between your limbs or desire a training variation.

- This exercise may be contraindicated if you have low-back pain or hyperextended knees.

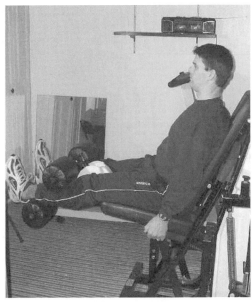
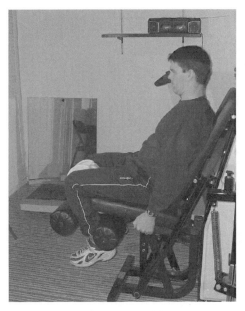

Start/Finish Position   *Mid-Range Position*

SEATED LEG CURL

Equipment Needed: resistance machine

Muscles Influenced: hamstrings

Suggested Repetitions: 10 - 15

Start/Finish Position: If possible, adjust the position of the lower leg pad and back pad (as described below in the training tips). Sit down on the seat pad and place your lower legs between the upper and lower leg pads. Position your knees so that they're approximately even with the axis of rotation of the machine. If the machine has handles, lightly grasp them (or grasp the seat pad).

Performance Description: Bring your heels as close to your hips as possible by pulling against the lower leg pad. Pause briefly in this mid-range position (your heels near your hips) and then lower the weight under control to the start/finish position (your legs fully extended) to ensure a sufficient stretch.

Training Tips:

- Adjust the position of the lower leg pad so that it's near the bottom part of your calves (just above your ankles) in the start/finish position.

- Adjust the position of the back pad so that your knees are approximately even with the axis of rotation of the machine.

- Keep your torso against the back pad as you perform this exercise – movement should only occur around your knee joints.

- The angle between your upper and lower legs should be about 90 degrees or less in the mid-range position. This could be deceiving if the seat pad is angled rather than parallel to the floor.

- Don't slam the weights together or bounce the movement arm against the machine between repetitions.

- You can do this exercise unilaterally (one limb at a time) if you have a leg or knee injury, a gross difference in the strength between your limbs or desire a training variation.

- Performing this exercise in the seated position produces less stress in the low-back region than performing it in the prone position.

- This exercise may be contraindicated if you have hyperextended knees.

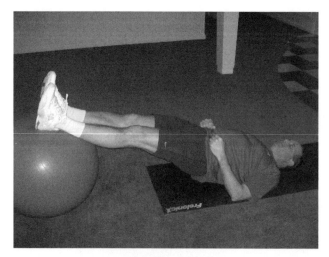
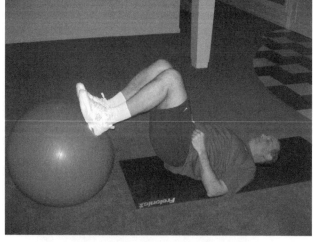

Start/Finish Position   *Mid-Range Position*

LEG CURL (stability ball)

Equipment Needed: stability ball

Muscles Influenced: hamstrings and erector spinae

Suggested Repetitions: 10 - 15

Start/Finish Position: Lie supine on the floor and place your lower legs on top of a stability ball. Straighten your legs and bring them together. Keep your shoulders on the floor and elevate your hips. Place your hands on your mid-section (or position your arms on the floor so that they are roughly perpendicular to your torso).

Performance Description: Bring your heels as close to your hips as possible by pulling against the ball. Pause briefly in this mid-range position (your heels near your hips) and then return under control to the start/finish position (your legs fully extended) to ensure a sufficient stretch.

Training Tips:

• Try to pull your heels as close to your hips as possible by using your hamstrings. Think about digging your heels into the ball and applying pressure down.

• Keep your shoulders on the floor and your hips elevated as you perform this exercise.

• This exercise is more difficult with your arms closer to your torso.

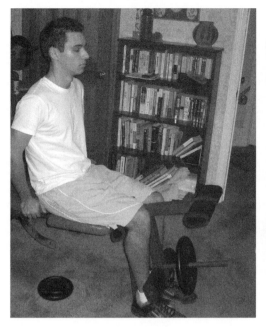 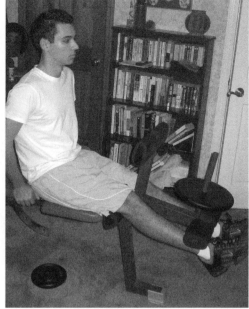

Start/Finish Position   *Mid-Range Position*

LEG EXTENSION

Equipment Needed: resistance machine

Muscles Influenced: quadriceps

Suggested Repetitions: 10 - 15

Start/Finish Position: If possible, adjust the position of the leg pad (as described below in the training tips). Sit down on the seat pad and place the backs of your knees against the end of it. Position your feet behind the leg pad. If the machine has handles, lightly grasp them (or grasp the seat pad).

Performance Description: Extend your lower legs as high as possible by pushing against the roller pads. Pause briefly in this mid-range position (your legs fully extended) and then return the weight under control to the start/finish position (your legs flexed) to obtain a proper stretch.

Training Tips:

- Adjust the position of the leg pad so that it's near the bottom part of your shins (just above your ankles) in the start/finish position. (Some machines have two leg pads rather than one.)

- Avoid throwing the weight by swinging your torso back and forth – movement should only occur around your knee joints.

- Attempt to raise the weight as high as possible in the mid-range position of every repetition to ensure that you're obtaining a maximal contraction of the target muscles throughout the duration of the exercise.

- Don't slam the weights together or bounce the movement arm against the machine between repetitions.

- You can do this exercise unilaterally (one limb at a time) if you have a leg or knee injury, a gross difference in the strength between your limbs or desire a training variation.

8

THE LOWER LEGS

Many important muscles are found in your lower legs. So, a strength-training program should address this area.

MUSCLES OF THE LOWER LEGS

The calves and the "dorsi flexors" are the two major muscle groups in your lower legs.

Calves

Your calves are made up of two important muscles – the gastrocnemius (or "gastroc") and soleus – that are located on the back of your lower legs. These two muscles have a common tendon of insertion (the Achilles tendon) and are jointly referred to as the "triceps surae" or, more simply, the "gastroc-soleus." Your soleus actually resides underneath your gastrocnemius and is used primarily when you extend your ankle while the angle between your upper and lower legs is about 90 degrees or less (such as in the seated position). The calves are involved in plantar flexion (extending your ankles or rising up on your toes). Your calves play a major role in running and jumping activities.

Dorsi Flexors

The front of your lower leg contains four muscles that are sometimes simply referred to as the "dorsi flexors." The largest of these muscles is the tibialis anterior. The dorsi flexors are primarily used in dorsi flexion (flexing your ankles). It's critical to strengthen your dorsi flexors as a safeguard against shin splints.

EXERCISES FOR THE LOWER LEGS

This chapter will describe and illustrate three exercises that you can perform for the muscles of your lower legs. These exercises are the seated calf raise, standing calf raise and dorsi flexion.

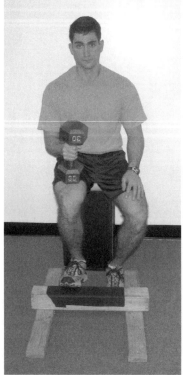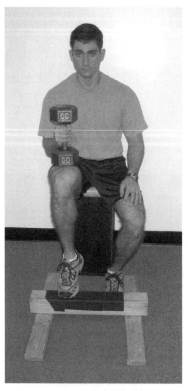

Start/Finish Position   *Mid-Range Position*

SEATED CALF RAISE

Equipment Needed: dumbbell, bench (or chair or stool) and step (or something similar)

Muscles Influenced: gastrocnemius (calves) and soleus (calves)

Suggested Repetitions: 10 - 15

Start/Finish Position: Sit down near the end of a bench (or a chair or stool). Place the ball of your right foot on the edge of a step (or something similar that's stable) and lower your heel. Position a dumbbell on the top of your right upper leg and hold it in place.

Performance Description: Rise up onto your toes as high as possible. Pause briefly in this mid-range position (your ankle extended) and then lower the weight under control to the start/finish position (your heel near the floor) to provide a proper stretch. After performing a set with your right ankle, repeat the exercise for the other side of your body.

Training Tips:

• The step is used to obtain a better stretch. If an unstable object is used instead of a stable one, another person can stand on the side of it to make it steadier.

• Avoid throwing the weight by using your arms or swinging your torso back and forth – movement should only occur around your ankle joint.

• Attempt to raise the weight as high as possible in the mid-range position of every repetition to ensure that you're obtaining a maximal contraction of the target muscles throughout the duration of the exercise.

• This exercise may be contraindicated if you have shin splints.

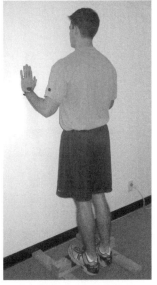
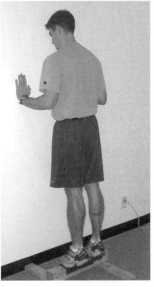

Start/Finish Position *Mid-Range Position*

STANDING CALF RAISE

Equipment Needed: step (or something similar)

Muscles Influenced: gastrocnemius (calves)

Suggested Repetitions: 10 - 15

Start/Finish Position: Stand on a step (or something similar that's stable). Hold onto the railing (or something similar or place your hands against a wall) to maintain your balance. Position the balls of your feet on the edge of the step and lower your heels.

Performance Description: Keep legs straight and rise up onto your toes as high as possible. Pause briefly in this mid-range position (your ankles extended) and then lower your body under control to the start/finish position (your heels near the floor) to ensure a proper stretch.

Training Tips:

- The step is used to obtain a better stretch. If an unstable object is used instead of a stable one, another person can stand on the side of it to make it steadier.

- It's natural for you to use your hips and legs as you perform this exercise. However, movement of your hips and legs shouldn't be excessive or used to raise your body – movement should only occur around your ankle joints.

- Traditionally, this exercise is done with a weight placed on the shoulders – either a barbell or the movement arm of a machine. This should be avoided whenever possible, however, because it compresses the spinal column.

- Attempt to raise your body as high as possible in the mid-range position of every repetition to ensure that you're obtaining a maximal contraction of the target muscles throughout the duration of the exercise.

- You can do this exercise unilaterally (one limb at a time) if you have a leg, knee or ankle injury, a gross difference in the strength between your limbs or desire a training variation.

- If you can do 15 repetitions or more with strict form using your bodyweight, you can increase the workload on your muscles by holding onto a dumbbell in one hand, doing the exercise unilaterally or performing the exercise with a slower speed of movement. (You can use wrist straps if you have difficulty in maintaining a grip on the dumbbell.)

- This exercise may be contraindicated if you have shin splints.

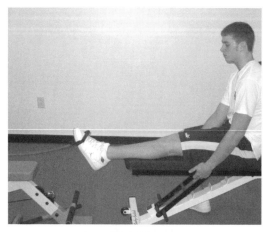 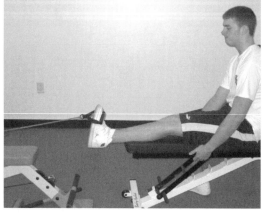

Start/Finish Position   *Mid-Range Position*

DORSI FLEXION

Equipment Needed: cable column, ankle/wrist strap and bench

Muscles Influenced: dorsi flexors

Suggested Repetitions: 10 - 15

Start/Finish Position: Adjust the position of the pulley so that it's near the bottom of the column and attach an ankle/wrist strap. Sit down near the end of the back pad of a bench and secure the ankle/wrist strap around your left foot between your toes and instep. Slide your hips back so that your left leg lies across the length of the pad and the weight you intend to lift is separated slightly from the rest of the weight stack. Position your left heel slightly over the end of the pad and point your left toes away from your body.

Performance Description: Keep your left leg flat on the pad and flex your left ankle as much as possible. Pause briefly in this mid-range position (your ankle flexed) and then lower the weight under control to the start/finish position (your ankle fully extended) to provide a proper stretch. After performing a set with your left ankle, repeat the exercise for the other side of your body.

Training Tips:

• Avoid throwing the weight by swinging your torso back and forth – movement should only occur around your ankle joint.

• Attempt to raise the weight as high as possible in the mid-range position of every repetition to ensure that you're obtaining a maximal contraction of the target muscles throughout the duration of the exercise.

• You can also perform this exercise with a resistance band/cord. The band/cord would be secured to an object that won't move. Otherwise, the exercise would be performed in the same fashion as described above.

• This exercise may be contraindicated if you have shin splints.

9

THE CHEST

The chest area – along with the upper back and shoulders – is one of the major muscle groups in your torso.

MUSCLES OF THE CHEST

The main muscles that surround your chest area are the pectoralis major and pectoralis minor. The pectoralis major is thick, flat and fan-shaped and the most superficial muscle of your chest wall. The pectoralis minor is thin, flat and triangular and positioned beneath your pectoralis major. The "pecs" pull your upper arms across your body. Like most of the muscles in the torso, your chest is involved in throwing and pushing movements.

EXERCISES FOR THE CHEST

This chapter will describe and illustrate seven exercises that you can perform for the muscles of your chest. The exercises are the bench press, incline press, decline press, dip, push-up, push-up (with a stability ball) and bent-arm fly.

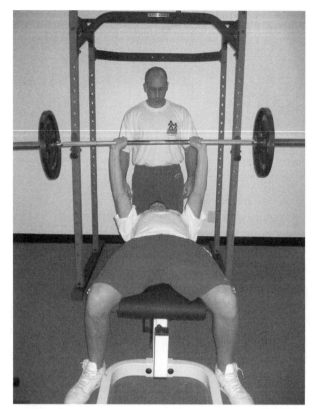

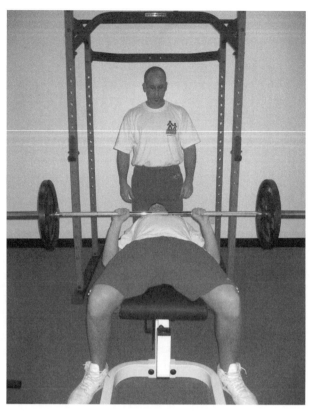

Start/Finish Position   *Mid-Range Position*

BENCH PRESS

Equipment Needed: barbell or dumbbells and bench

Muscles Influenced: chest, anterior deltoids and triceps

Suggested Repetitions: 6 - 12

Start/Finish Position: Lie down on the back pad of a bench and place your feet flat on the floor. Grasp the bar and spread your hands slightly wider than shoulder-width apart. Lift the bar out of the uprights or have another person (a "spotter") give you assistance. Keep your arms almost fully extended (that is, without "locking" your elbows).

Performance Description: Lower the bar under control until it touches the middle part of your chest. Without bouncing the weight off your chest, push the bar up to the start/finish position (your arms almost fully extended).

Training Tips:

- For reasons of safety, you shouldn't perform this exercise without a spotter.
- You shouldn't use an excessively wide grip since this will reduce your range of motion.
- Keep your hips flat on the pad and your feet flat on the floor as you perform this exercise. If you have low-back pain, you can place your feet on the end of the pad, a chair or a stool. This will flatten your lumbar area against the pad and reduce the stress in your low-back region.
- You shouldn't "lock" or "snap" your elbows in the start/finish position of a repetition. This removes the load from the target muscles and may hyperextend your elbows.
- Don't bounce the weight off your chest between repetitions.
- You should move the bar upward and backward as you press the weight.
- You can also perform this exercise with dumbbells in the same fashion as described above.

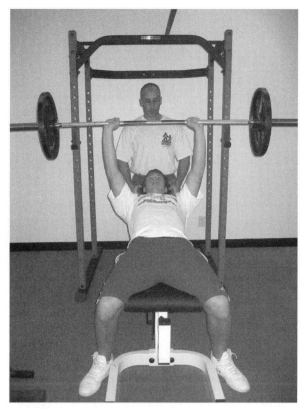 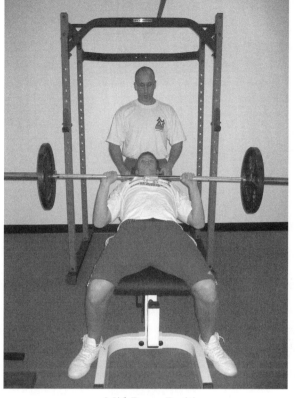

Start/Finish Position   *Mid-Range Position*

INCLINE PRESS

Equipment Needed: barbell or dumbbells and adjustable bench

Muscles Influenced: chest (upper portion), anterior deltoids and triceps

Suggested Repetitions: 6 - 12

Start/Finish Position: Adjust the position of a bench so that the back pad is inclined at about a 45-degree angle. Sit down on the seat pad, lie back against the back pad and place your feet flat on the floor. Grasp the bar and space your hands slightly wider than shoulder-width apart. Lift the bar out of the uprights or have another person (a "spotter") give you assistance. Keep your arms almost fully extended (that is, without "locking" your elbows).

Performance Description: Lower the bar under control until it touches the upper part of your chest (near your collarbones). Without bouncing the weight off your chest, push the bar up to the start/finish position (your arms almost fully extended).

Training Tips:

- For reasons of safety, you shouldn't perform this exercise without a spotter.
- You shouldn't use an excessively wide grip since this will reduce your range of motion.
- Keep your hips flat on the seat pad and your feet flat on the floor as you perform this exercise. If you have low-back pain, you can place your feet on a chair or a stool. This will flatten your lumbar area against the back pad and reduce the stress in your low-back region.
- You shouldn't "lock" or "snap" your elbows in the start/finish position of a repetition. This removes the load from the target muscles and may hyperextend your elbows.
- Don't bounce the weight off your chest between repetitions.
- You should move the bar upward and backward as you press the weight.
- You can also perform this exercise with dumbbells in the same fashion as described above.

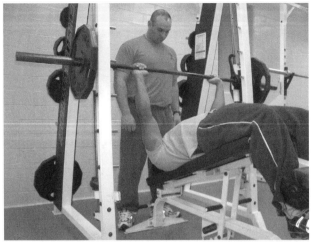
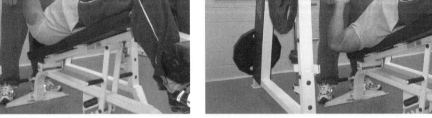

| *Start/Finish Position* | *Mid-Range Position* |

DECLINE PRESS

Equipment Needed: barbell or dumbbells and adjustable bench

Muscles Influenced: chest (lower portion), anterior deltoid and triceps

Suggested Repetitions: 6 - 12

Start/Finish Position: Adjust the position of a bench so that the back pad is declined at about a 30-degree angle. Lie down on the back pad and place your lower legs behind the leg pads. Grasp the bar and space your hands slightly wider than shoulder-width apart. Lift the bar out of the up-rights or have another person (a "spotter") give you assistance. Keep your arms almost fully extended (that is, without "locking" your elbows).

Performance Description: Lower the bar under control until it touches the lower part of your chest (near the tip of your breastbone). Without bouncing the weight off your chest, push the bar up to the start/finish position (your arms almost fully extended).

Training Tips:

- For reasons of safety, you shouldn't perform this exercise without a spotter.
- You shouldn't use an excessively wide grip since this will reduce your range of motion.
- Keep your hips flat on the pad as you perform this exercise.
- You shouldn't "lock" or "snap" your elbows in the start/finish position of a repetition. This removes the load from the target muscles and may hyperextend your elbows.
- Don't bounce the weight off your chest between repetitions.
- You should move the bar upward and backward as you press the weight.
- You can also perform this exercise with dumbbells in the same fashion as described above.

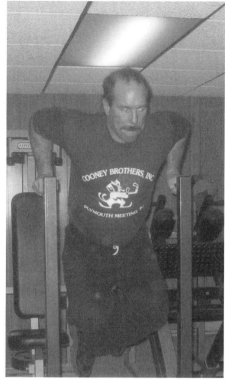
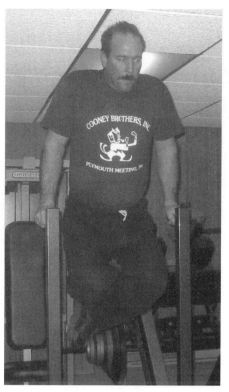

Start/Finish Position   *Mid-Range Position*

DIP

Equipment Needed: dip bars/handles

Muscles Influenced: chest (lower portion), anterior deltoids and triceps

Suggested Repetitions: 6 - 12

Start/Finish Position: Grasp the bars/handles with a "parallel grip" (your palms facing each other). Bend your arms such that your upper arms are roughly parallel to the floor. Lift your feet off the floor, bend your knees and cross your ankles.

Performance Description: Push yourself up until your arms are almost fully extended (that is, without "locking" your elbows). Pause briefly in this mid-range position (your arms almost fully extended) and then lower your body under control to the start/finish position (your arms flexed) to obtain a sufficient stretch.

Training Tips:

- Avoid swinging your body back and forth as you perform this exercise – movement should only occur around your shoulder and elbow joints.

- You shouldn't "lock" or "snap" your elbows in the mid-range position of a repetition. This removes the load from the target muscles and may hyperextend your elbows.

- If you cannot do 6 repetitions with strict form using your bodyweight, you can exercise the same muscles in a similar fashion by performing the decline press.

- If you can do 12 repetitions or more with strict form using your bodyweight, you can increase the workload on your muscles by attaching extra weight to your waist or performing the exercise with a slower speed of movement.

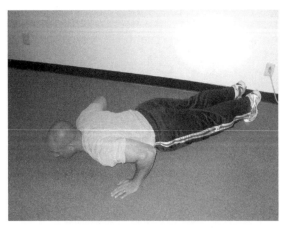 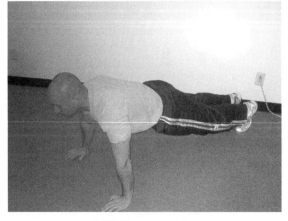

Start/Finish Position   *Mid-Range Position*

PUSH-UP

Equipment Needed: none

Muscles Influenced: chest, anterior deltoids and triceps

Suggested Repetitions: 6 - 12

Start/Finish Position: Lie prone on the floor, straighten your legs and curl your toes under your feet. Place your palms on the floor and spread your hands slightly wider than shoulder-width apart.

Performance Description: Push your body up until your arms are almost fully extended (that is, without "locking" your elbows). Pause briefly in this mid-range position (your arms almost fully extended) and then lower your body under control to the start/finish position (your chest touching the floor) to obtain a sufficient stretch.

Training Tips:

- You shouldn't use an excessively wide hand position since this will reduce your range of motion.
- Avoid arching your lower back as you perform this exercise – your torso should remain aligned with your lower body.
- You shouldn't "lock" or "snap" your elbows in the mid-range position of a repetition. This removes the load from the target muscles and may hyperextend your elbows.
- If you cannot do 6 repetitions with strict form using your bodyweight, you can increase your biomechanical leverage by performing this exercise in the kneeling position.
- If you can do 12 repetitions or more with strict form using your bodyweight, you can increase the workload on your muscles by elevating your feet onto a bench, chair or stool or performing the exercise with a slower speed of movement. (Elevating your feet will change the emphasis of the exercise to the upper portion of your chest.)

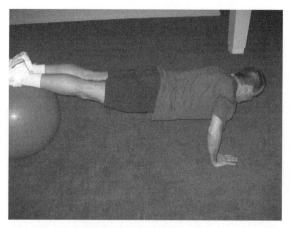 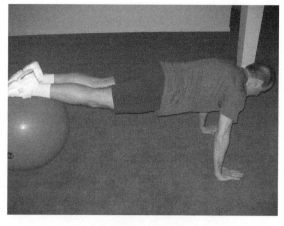

Start/Finish Position   *Mid-Range Position*

PUSH-UP (stability ball)

Equipment Needed: stability ball

Muscles Influenced: chest (upper portion), anterior deltoids and triceps

Suggested Repetitions: 6 - 12

Start/Finish Position: Lie prone on the floor, straighten your legs and position your lower legs on a stability ball. Place your palms on the floor and spread your hands slightly wider than shoulder-width apart.

Performance Description: Push your body up until your arms are almost fully extended (that is, without "locking" your elbows). Pause briefly in this mid-range position (your arms almost fully extended) and then lower your body under control to the start/finish position (your chest touching the floor) to obtain a sufficient stretch.

Training Tips:

• You shouldn't use an excessively wide hand position since this will reduce your range of motion.

• Avoid arching your lower back as you perform this exercise – your torso should remain aligned with your lower body.

• You shouldn't "lock" or "snap" your elbows in the mid-range position of a repetition. This removes the load from the target muscles and may hyperextend your elbows.

• If you cannot do this exercise – or have a very difficult time doing so – you can progress to it by first doing push-ups with your feet on something more stable such as a bench, chair or stool.

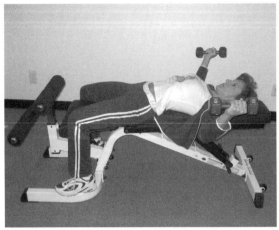

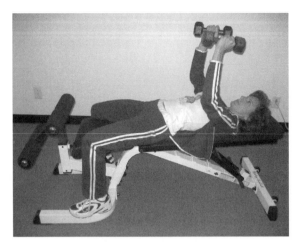

| Start/Finish Position | Mid-Range Position |

BENT-ARM FLY

Equipment Needed: dumbbells and bench

Muscles Influenced: chest and anterior deltoids

Suggested Repetitions: 6 - 12

Start/Finish Position: Sit down near the end of the back pad of a bench, reach down and grasp two dumbbells. Lift the dumbbells, lie down on the pad and place your feet flat on the floor. Position the dumbbells on both sides of your torso so that they're even with your chest. Point your palms toward each other and move the dumbbells up and away from your chest until the angle between your upper and lower arms is about 90 degrees.

Performance Description: Without significantly changing the angle between your upper and lower arms, bring the dumbbells together above your chest. Pause briefly in this mid-range position (the dumbbells directly over your chest) and then return the weights under control to the start/finish position (the dumbbells away from each other) to obtain a sufficient stretch.

Training Tips:

• Maintain about a 90-degree angle between your upper and lower arms as you raise and lower the dumbbells. (Imagine that you're hugging a tree.) If you straighten your arms as you raise the dumbbells, you'll change the exercise from a bent-arm fly into a bench press.

• Keep your hips flat on the pad and your feet flat on the floor as you perform this exercise. If you have low-back pain, you can place your feet on the end of the pad, a chair or stool. This will flatten your lumbar area against the pad and reduce the stress in your low-back region.

10

THE UPPER BACK

The upper back – along with the chest and shoulders – is one of the major muscle groups in your torso.

MUSCLES OF THE UPPER BACK

The latissimus dorsi is a long, broad muscle that comprises most of your upper back. As a matter of fact, the "lats" are the largest muscle in your torso. Its primary function is to pull your upper arms backward and downward. The muscle is particularly important in assorted pulling movements and climbing skills. In addition, developing the latissimus dorsi is necessary to provide muscular balance between your upper back and chest.

EXERCISES FOR THE UPPER BACK

This chapter will describe and illustrate seven exercises that you can perform for the muscles of your upper back. The exercises are the underhand lat pulldown, overhand lat pulldown, chin, pull-up, seated row, bent-over row and pullover.

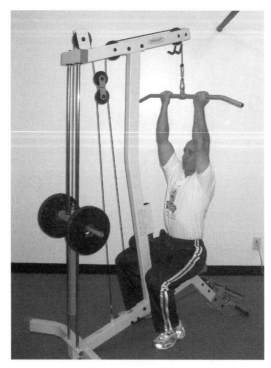 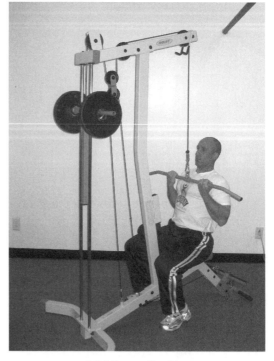

Start/Finish Position   *Mid-Range Position*

UNDERHAND LAT PULLDOWN

Equipment Needed: cable column and bar

Muscles Influenced: upper back ("lats"), biceps and forearms

Suggested Repetitions: 6 - 12

Start/Finish Position: Adjust the position of the pulley so that it's near the top of the column and attach a bar. Reach up, grasp the bar with your palms facing you and space your hands approximately shoulder-width apart. Sit down on the seat pad, place your upper legs under the roller pads (if provided) and lean back slightly.

Performance Description: Pull the bar down to your upper chest and draw your elbows backward. Pause briefly in this mid-range position (your arms flexed) and then return the weight under control to the start/finish position (your arms fully extended) to obtain a proper stretch.

Training Tips:

- Avoid swinging your torso back and forth as you perform this exercise – movement should only occur around your shoulder and elbow joints.

- Touching the bar to your upper chest rather than your chin will increase your range of motion. Drawing your elbows backward in the mid-range position will increase the workload performed by your upper back.

- You can do this exercise unilaterally (one limb at a time) if you have a shoulder or arm injury, a gross difference in the strength between your limbs or desire a training variation. (To do the exercise unilaterally requires a handle instead of a bar.)

- You can use wrist straps if you have difficulty in maintaining your grip on the bar.

- This exercise may be contraindicated if you have hyperextended elbows.

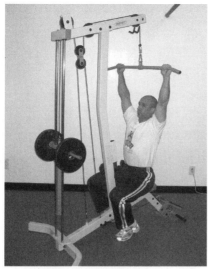
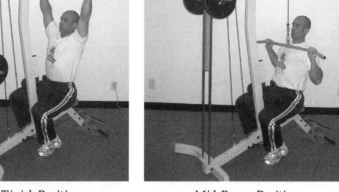

Start/Finish Position   *Mid-Range Position*

OVERHAND LAT PULLDOWN

Equipment Needed: cable column and bar

Muscles Influenced: upper back ("lats"), biceps and forearms

Suggested Repetitions: 6 - 12

Start/Finish Position: Adjust the position of the pulley so that it's near the top of the column and attach a bar. Reach up, grasp the bar with your palms facing away from you and space your hands several inches wider than shoulder-width apart. Sit down on the seat pad, place your upper legs under the roller pads (if provided) and lean back slightly.

Performance Description: Pull the bar down to your upper chest and draw your elbows downward. Pause briefly in this mid-range position (your arms flexed) and then lower the weight under control to the start/finish position (your arms fully extended) to obtain an adequate stretch.

Training Tips:

- Avoid swinging your torso back and forth as you perform this exercise – movement should only occur around your shoulder and elbow joints.

- You shouldn't use an excessively wide grip since this will reduce your range of motion.

- Touching the bar to your upper chest rather than your chin will increase your range of motion. Drawing your elbows backward in the mid-range position will increase the workload performed by your upper back.

- You can do this exercise unilaterally (one limb at a time) if you have a shoulder or arm injury, a gross difference in the strength between your limbs or desire a training variation. (To do the exercise unilaterally requires a handle instead of a bar.)

- Performing a lat pulldown with an overhand grip (your palms facing away from you) isn't as biomechanically efficient as doing it with an underhand grip (your palms facing toward you). But this exercise is still quite productive when performed with an overhand grip in the manner described above.

- You can use wrist straps if you have difficulty in maintaining your grip on the bar.

- You can also perform this exercise by pulling the bar down so that it travels behind your head to the base of your neck. However, this exercise may be contraindicated if you have shoulder-impingement syndrome. This exercise may also be contraindicated if you have hyperextended elbows.

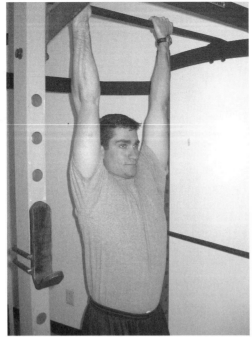
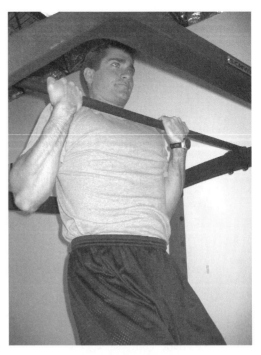

Start/Finish Position   Mid-Range Position

CHIN

Equipment Needed: chin/pull-up bar

Muscles Influenced: upper back ("lats"), biceps and forearms

Suggested Repetitions: 6 - 12

Start/Finish Position: Reach up, grasp a chin/pull-up bar with your palms facing you and space your hands approximately shoulder-width apart. Bring your body to a "dead hang" and cross your ankles.

Performance Description: Pull your body up so that your upper chest touches the bar and draw your elbows backward. Pause briefly in this mid-range position (your arms flexed) and then lower your body under control back to the start/finish position (your arms fully extended) to obtain a proper stretch.

Training Tips:

- Avoid swinging your body back and forth as you perform this exercise – movement should only occur around your shoulder and elbow joints.

- Touching your upper chest to the bar rather than your chin will increase your range of motion. Drawing your elbows backward in the mid-range position will increase the workload performed by your upper back.

- If you cannot do 6 repetitions with strict form using your bodyweight, you can exercise the same muscles in a similar fashion by performing the underhand lat pulldown.

- If you can do 12 repetitions or more with strict form using your bodyweight, you can increase the workload on your muscles by attaching extra weight to your waist or performing the exercise with a slower speed of movement.

- You can use wrist straps if you have difficulty in maintaining your grip on the bar.

- This exercise may be contraindicated if you have hyperextended elbows.

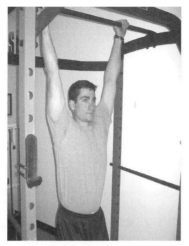 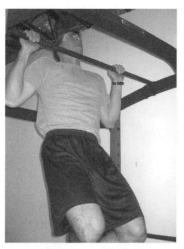

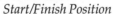

Start/Finish Position   *Mid-Range Position*

PULL-UP

Equipment Needed: chin/pull-up bar

Muscles Influenced: upper back ("lats"), biceps and forearms

Suggested Repetitions: 6 - 12

Start/Finish Position: Reach up, grasp a chin/pull-up bar with your palms facing away from you and space your hands several inches wider than shoulder-width apart. Bring your body to a "dead hang" and cross your ankles.

Performance Description: Pull your body up so that your upper chest touches the bar and draw your elbows backward. Pause briefly in this mid-range position (your arms flexed) and then lower your body under control to the start/finish position (your arms fully extended) to obtain an adequate stretch.

Training Tips:

- Avoid swinging your body back and forth as you perform this exercise – movement should only occur around your shoulder and elbow joints.

- You shouldn't use an excessively wide grip since this will reduce your range of motion.

- Touching your upper chest to the bar rather than your chin will increase your range of motion. Drawing your elbows backward in the mid-range position will increase the workload performed by your upper back.

- If you cannot do 6 repetitions with strict form using your bodyweight, you can exercise the same muscles in a similar fashion by performing the overhand lat pulldown.

- If you can do 12 repetitions or more with strict form using your bodyweight, you can increase the workload on your muscles by attaching extra weight to your waist or performing the exercise with a slower speed of movement.

- Performing a pull-up with an overhand grip (your palms facing away from you) isn't as biomechanically efficient as doing a chin with an underhand grip (your palms facing toward you). But this exercise is still quite productive when performed in the manner described above.

- You can use wrist straps if you have difficulty in maintaining your grip on the bar.

- You can also perform this exercise by pulling your body up so that the bar travels behind your head to the base of your neck. However, this may be contraindicated if you have shoulder-impingement syndrome. This exercise may also be contraindicated if you have hyperextended elbows.

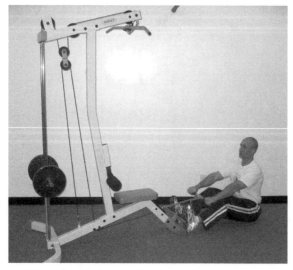
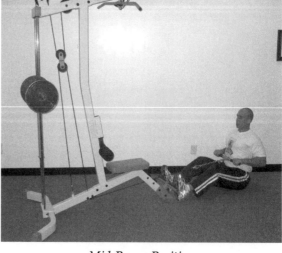

Start/Finish Position   *Mid-Range Position*

SEATED ROW

Equipment Needed: cable column and bar

Muscles Influenced: upper back ("lats"), biceps and forearms

Suggested Repetitions: 6 - 12

Start/Finish Position: Adjust the position of the pulley so that it's near the bottom of the column and attach a bar. Sit down on the floor, grasp the bar with your palms facing down and space your hands approximately shoulder-width apart. Straighten your legs but maintain a slight bend at your knees and sit upright. Adjust the position of your legs so that the weight you intend to lift is separated slightly from the rest of the weight stack. Lean back slightly.

Performance Description: Keep your upper arms close to your torso and pull the bar to your mid-section. Pause briefly in this mid-range position (your arms flexed) and then lower the weight under control to the start/finish position (your arms fully extended) to ensure a sufficient stretch.

Training Tips:

• It's natural for you to change the position of your torso as you perform this exercise. However, movement of your torso shouldn't be excessive or used to throw the weight – movement should only occur around your shoulder and elbow joints.

• Don't slam the weights together between repetitions.

• You can do this exercise unilaterally (one limb at a time) if you have a shoulder or arm injury, a gross difference in the strength between your limbs or desire a training variation. (To do the exercise unilaterally requires a handle instead of a bar.)

• You can also perform this exercise with an underhand grip (your palms facing up) in the manner described above.

• You can use wrist straps if you have difficulty in maintaining your grip on the handles.

• This exercise may be contraindicated if you have hyperextended elbows.

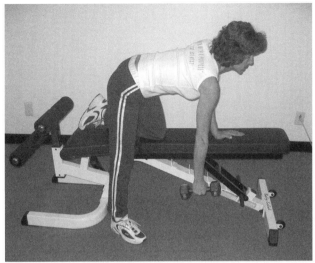
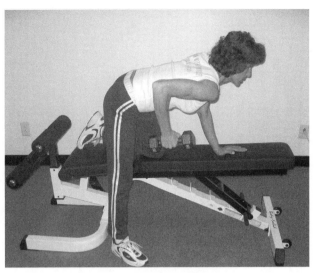

Start/Finish Position   *Mid-Range Position*

BENT-OVER ROW

Equipment Needed: dumbbell and bench

Muscles Influenced: upper back ("lats"), biceps and forearms

Suggested Repetitions: 6 - 12

Start/Finish Position: Place your left hand and left knee on the back pad of a bench. Position your right foot on the floor at a comfortable distance from the bench. Reach down and grasp a dumbbell with your right hand. Lift the dumbbell slightly off the floor and straighten your right arm. Your right palm should be facing the bench.

Performance Description: Keep your upper arm close to your torso and pull the dumbbell up to your right shoulder. Pause briefly in this mid-range position (your arm flexed) and then return the dumbbell under control to the start/finish position (your arm fully extended) to ensure an adequate stretch. After performing a set with your right arm, repeat the exercise for the other side of your body (with your right hand and right knee on the back pad for support).

Training Tips:

- It's natural for you to change the position of your shoulder as you perform this exercise. However, movement of your shoulder shouldn't be excessive or used to throw the dumbbell – movement should only occur around your shoulder and elbow joints.

- You can also do this exercise with your upper arm positioned farther away from your torso. Keep in mind, however, that this will produce a greater involvement of your posterior deltoid and trapezius. In this case, your upper arm would be almost perpendicular to your torso in the mid-range position and your palm would be facing backward slightly.

- You can use wrist straps if you have difficulty in maintaining your grip on the dumbbell.

- This exercise may be contraindicated if you have a hyperextended elbow.

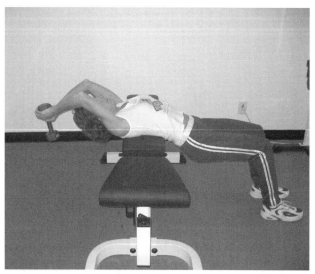
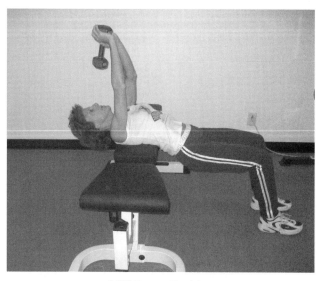

Start/Finish Position   *Mid-Range Position*

PULLOVER

Equipment Needed: dumbbell or barbell and bench

Muscles Influenced: upper back ("lats")

Suggested Repetitions: 6 - 12

Start/Finish Position: Sit down near the middle of the back pad of a bench, reach down and grasp a dumbbell. Lift the dumbbell and lie down across the pad. Position your shoulder blades such that your torso is perpendicular to the length of the pad and place your feet flat on the floor. Hold the dumbbell by placing your palms against the innermost plate (not the handle). Keep your arms relatively straight and lower the dumbbell toward the floor so that your elbows are near or slightly past your head. (Another person may be needed to position a heavy weight.)

Performance Description: Without bending your arms, pull the dumbbell directly over your head. Pause briefly in this mid-range position (the dumbbell directly over your head) and then lower the dumbbell under control to the start/finish position (the dumbbell near the floor) to ensure an adequate stretch.

Training Tips:

• You can also perform this exercise with a barbell (spacing your hands about 4 - 6 inches apart).

• This exercise may be contraindicated if you have low-back pain or shoulder-impingement syndrome.

11

THE SHOULDERS

The shoulders – along with the chest and upper back – are one of the major muscle groups in your torso.

MUSCLES OF THE SHOULDERS

Your shoulders are made up of 11 muscles. The primary muscles are the deltoids, the so-called "rotator cuff" and the trapezius.

Deltoids

The most important muscles in your shoulders are the deltoids. Your "delts" are actually composed of three separate parts (or "heads"). The anterior deltoid is found on the front of your shoulder and is used to raise your upper arm forward; the middle deltoid is located on the side of your shoulder and is used to raise your upper arm sideways; and the posterior deltoid is found on the back of your shoulder and is used to draw your upper arm backward.

Rotator Cuff

Several other deep muscles of the shoulder are sometimes referred to as the "internal rotators" (the subscapularis and teres major) and the "external rotators" (the infraspinatus and teres minor). In addition to performing rotation, these muscles are also largely responsible for maintaining the integrity of your shoulder joint and in preventing shoulder impingement. Along with the muscles of the chest, strong shoulders are a vital part of throwing skills and pushing movements.

Trapezius

The trapezius is a kite-shaped (or trapezoid-shaped) muscle that covers the uppermost region of your back and the posterior section of your neck. The primary functions of your "traps" are shoulder elevation (shrugging your shoulders as if to say, "I don't know"), scapulae adduction ("pinching" your shoulder blades together) and neck extension (bringing your head backward). The trapezius is often considered part of the neck musculature.

EXERCISES FOR THE SHOULDERS

This chapter will describe and illustrate 14 exercises that you can perform for the muscles of your shoulders. These exercises are the seated press, lateral raise, lateral raise (with a cable column), front raise, front raise (with a cable column), bent-over raise, bent-over raise (with a cable column), external rotation, external rotation (with a cable column), internal rotation, internal rotation (with a cable column), upright row, shoulder shrug and scapula retraction.

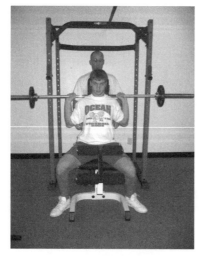
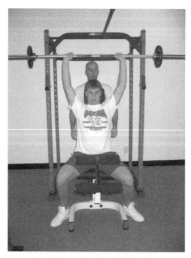

Start/Finish Position   *Mid-Range Position*

SEATED PRESS

Equipment Needed: barbell or dumbbells and bench (or chair or stool)

Muscles Influenced: anterior deltoids and triceps

Suggested Repetitions: 6 - 12

Start/Finish Position: Reach down and grasp a bar with your palms facing you. Stand upright by straightening your legs and torso. Raise the bar above your head and then lower it behind your neck. Position the bar on the upper part of your trapezius. (Another person may be needed to position a heavy weight.) Sit down on the seat pad of a bench (or a chair or stool) and lean back against the back pad (if one is provided). Place your feet flat on the floor and spread your hands slightly wider than shoulder-width apart.

Performance Description: Push the bar up until your arms are almost fully extended (that is, without "locking" your elbows). Pause briefly in this mid-range position (your arms almost fully extended) and then return the weight under control to the start/finish position (your arms flexed) to provide a proper stretch.

Training Tips:

• For reasons of safety, you shouldn't perform this exercise without a spotter.

• You shouldn't use an excessively wide grip since this will reduce your range of motion.

• Keep your hips flat on the seat pad, your torso against the back pad (if one is provided) and your feet flat on the floor as you perform this exercise. If you have low-back pain, you can place your feet on a chair or a stool. This will flatten your lumbar area against the back pad and reduce the stress in your low-back region.

• You shouldn't "lock" or "snap" your elbows in the mid-range position of a repetition. This removes the load from the target muscles and may hyperextend your elbows.

• You can also perform this exercise with dumbbells in the same manner as described above.

• You can do this exercise unilaterally (one limb at a time) if you have a shoulder or an arm injury, a gross difference in the strength between your limbs or desire a training variation. (To do the exercise unilaterally requires a dumbbell instead of a barbell.)

• This exercise may be contraindicated if you have shoulder-impingement syndrome. In this case, however, raising and lowering the bar in front of your head rather than behind it will reduce the stress on an impinged shoulder. This exercise may also be contraindicated if you have low-back pain.

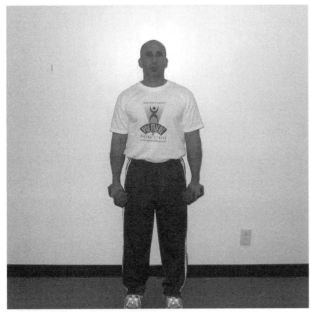
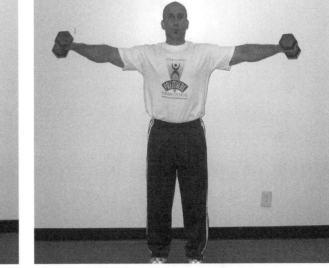

Start/Finish Position   *Mid-Range Position*

LATERAL RAISE

Equipment Needed: dumbbells

Muscles Influenced: middle deltoids and trapezius (upper portion)

Suggested Repetitions: 6 - 12

Start/Finish Position: Reach down and grasp a dumbbell in each hand. Stand upright by straightening your legs and torso. Hold the dumbbells against the sides of your body with your palms facing your legs. Straighten your arms and spread your feet about shoulder-width apart.

Performance Description: Keep your arms fairly straight and raise the dumbbells sideways until your arms are parallel to the floor. Pause briefly in this mid-range position (your arms parallel to the floor) and then lower the dumbbells under control to the start/finish position (your arms at your sides) to ensure an adequate stretch.

Training Tips:

- Avoid throwing the dumbbells by using your legs or swinging your torso back and forth – movement should only occur around your shoulder joints.

- You shouldn't raise your arms beyond a point that's parallel to the floor.

- Your palms should be facing the floor in the mid-range position.

- You can do this exercise unilaterally (one limb at a time) if you have a shoulder or an arm injury, a gross difference in the strength between your limbs or desire a training variation.

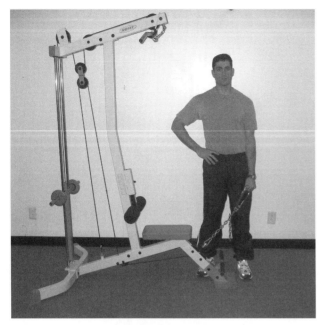 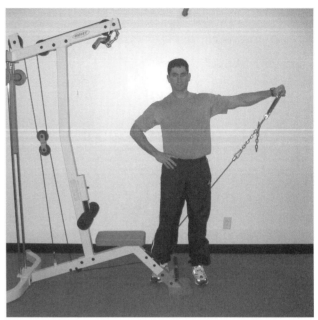

Start/Finish Position   *Mid-Range Position*

LATERAL RAISE (cable column)

Equipment Needed: cable column and handle

Muscles Influenced: middle deltoid and trapezius (upper portion)

Suggested Repetitions: 6 - 12

Start/Finish Position: Adjust the position of the pulley so that it's near the bottom of the column and attach a handle. Reach down and grasp the handle with your left hand. Stand upright by straightening your legs and torso. Turn your feet so that your right side is facing the machine. Slide your feet away from the machine so that the weight you intend to lift is separated slightly from the rest of the weight stack. Position your right hand on your right hip (or allow your right arm to hang straight down). Hold the handle near the left side of your body with your palm facing your leg. Straighten your left arm and spread your feet about shoulder-width apart.

Performance Description: Keep your arm fairly straight and raise the handle sideways until your arm is parallel to the floor. Pause briefly in this mid-range position (your arm parallel to the floor) and then lower the weight under control to the start/finish position (your arm at your side) to ensure an adequate stretch. After performing a set with your left arm, repeat the exercise for the other side of your body.

Training Tips:

• Avoid throwing the weight by using your legs or swinging your torso back and forth – movement should only occur around your shoulder joint.

• You shouldn't raise your arm beyond a point that's parallel to the floor.

• Your palm should be facing the floor in the mid-range position.

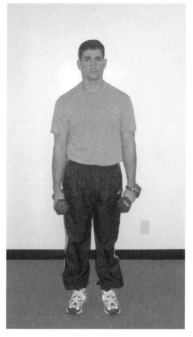
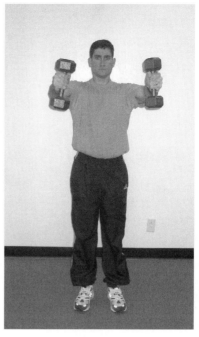

Start/Finish Position   *Mid-Range Position*

FRONT RAISE

Equipment Needed: dumbbells

Muscle Influenced: anterior deltoids

Suggested Repetitions: 6 - 12

Start/Finish Position: Reach down and grasp a dumbbell in each hand. Stand upright by straightening your legs and torso. Hold the dumbbells against the sides of your body with your palms facing your legs. Straighten your arms and spread your feet about shoulder-width apart (or place one foot slightly in front of the other).

Performance Description: Keep your arms fairly straight and raise the dumbbells forward until your arms are parallel to the floor. Pause briefly in this mid-range position (your arms parallel to the floor) and then return the dumbbells under control to the start/finish position (your arms at your sides) to obtain a proper stretch.

Training Tips:

• Avoid throwing the dumbbells by using your legs or swinging your torso back and forth – movement should only occur around your shoulder joints.

• You shouldn't raise your arms beyond a point that's parallel to the floor.

• Your palms should be facing each other in the mid-range position.

• You can do this exercise unilaterally (one limb at a time) if you have a shoulder or an arm injury, a gross difference in the strength between your limbs or desire a training variation.

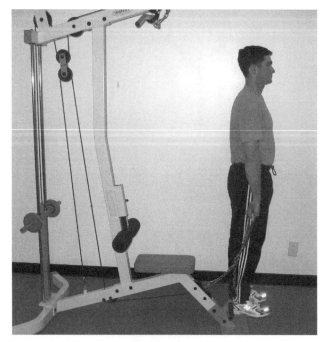
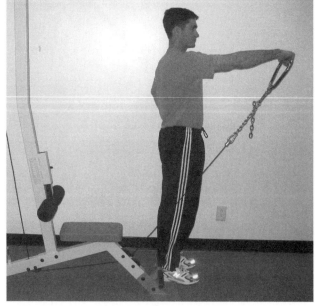

Start/Finish Position   *Mid-Range Position*

FRONT RAISE (cable column)

Equipment Needed: cable column and handle

Muscle Influenced: anterior deltoid

Suggested Repetitions: 6 - 12

Start/Finish Position: Adjust the position of the pulley so that it's near the bottom of the column and attach a handle. Reach down and grasp the handle with your right hand. Stand upright by straightening your legs and torso. Turn your feet so that your back is facing the machine. Slide your feet away from the machine so that the weight you intend to lift is separated slightly from the rest of the weight stack. Position your left hand on your left hip (or allow your left arm to hang straight down). Hold the handle near the right side of your body with your palm facing the machine. Straighten your right arm and spread your feet about shoulder-width apart (or place your left foot slightly in front of your right foot).

Performance Description: Keep your arm fairly straight and raise the handle forward until your arm is parallel to the floor. Pause briefly in this mid-range position (your arm parallel to the floor) and then return the weight under control to the start/finish position (your arm at your side) to obtain a proper stretch. After performing a set with your right arm, repeat the exercise for the other side of your body (and, if you've chosen to stagger your stance, with your right foot slightly in front of your left foot).

Training Tips:

• Avoid throwing the weight by using your legs or swinging your torso back and forth – movement should only occur around your shoulder joint.

• You shouldn't raise your arm beyond a point that's parallel to the floor.

• Your palm should be facing the floor in the mid-range position.

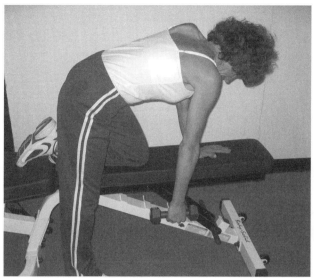
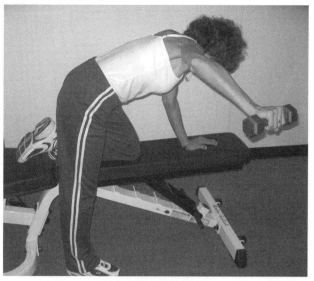

Start/Finish Position   *Mid-Range Position*

BENT-OVER RAISE

Equipment Needed: dumbbell and bench

Muscle Influenced: posterior deltoid and trapezius (middle portion)

Suggested Repetitions: 6 - 12

Start/Finish Position: Place your left hand and left knee on the back pad of a bench. Position your right foot on the floor at a comfortable distance from the bench. Reach down and grasp a dumbbell with your right hand. Lift the dumbbell slightly off the floor and straighten your right arm. Your right palm should be facing the bench.

Performance Description: Keep your arm fairly straight and raise the dumbbell sideways until your arm is parallel to the floor. Pause briefly in this mid-range position (your arm parallel to the floor) and then return the dumbbell under control to the start/finish position (your arm near the bench) to obtain a proper stretch. After performing a set with your right arm, repeat the exercise for the other side of your body (with your right hand and right knee on the back pad for support).

Training Tips:

• It's natural for you to change the position of your torso as you perform this exercise. However, movement of your torso shouldn't be excessive or used to throw the dumbbell – movement should only occur around your shoulder joint.

• You shouldn't raise your arm beyond a point that's parallel to the floor.

• Your palm should be facing the floor and your upper arm should be perpendicular to your torso in the mid-range position.

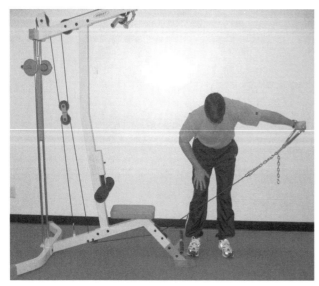

Start/Finish Position

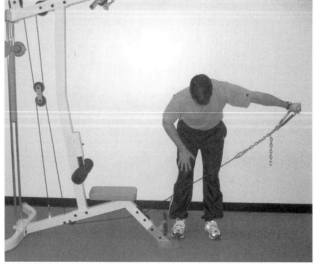

Mid-Range Position

BENT-OVER RAISE (cable column)

Equipment Needed: cable column and handle

Muscles Influenced: posterior deltoid and trapezius (middle portion)

Suggested Repetitions: 6 - 12

Start/Finish Position: Adjust the position of the pulley so that it's near the bottom of the column and attach a handle. Reach down and grasp the handle with your left hand. Stand upright by straightening your legs and torso. Turn your feet so that your right side is facing the machine. Slide your feet away from the machine so that the weight you intend to lift is separated slightly from the rest of the weight stack. Bend your hips and legs and position your right hand on your right thigh just above your knee. Hold the handle so that your left arm is across your torso. Straighten your left arm and spread your feet about shoulder-width apart.

Performance Description: Keep your left arm fairly straight and raise the handle sideways until your arm is parallel to the floor. Pause briefly in this mid-range position (your arm parallel to the floor) and then return the weight under control to the start/finish position (your arm across your torso) to obtain a proper stretch. After performing a set with your left arm, repeat the exercise for the other side of your body (with your left hand on your left thigh just above your knee).

Training Tips:

• It's natural for you to change the position of your torso as you perform this exercise. However, movement of your torso shouldn't be excessive or used to throw the weight – movement should only occur around your shoulder joint.

• You shouldn't raise your arm beyond a point that's parallel to the floor.

• Your palm should be facing the floor and your upper arm should be perpendicular to your torso in the mid-range position.

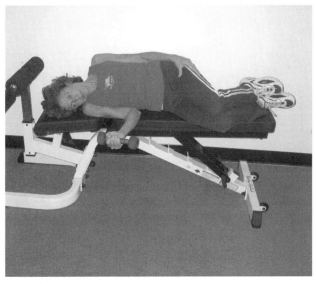 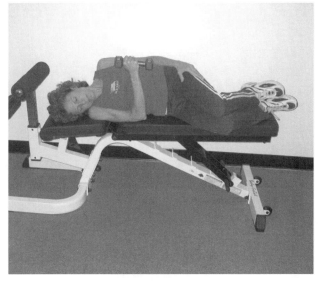

Start/Finish Position   *Mid-Range Position*

INTERNAL ROTATION

Equipment Needed: dumbbell and bench

Muscles Influenced: internal rotators

Suggested Repetitions: 6 - 12

Start/Finish Position: Grasp a dumbbell with your right hand, lie down on the back pad of a bench on your right side and draw your knees toward your torso. Position your right elbow just in front of your torso and bend your right arm so that the angle between your upper and lower arms is about 90 degrees. Point your right palm upward.

Performance Description: Without moving your elbow or changing the angle of your arm, pull the dumbbell to your mid-section. Pause briefly in this mid-range position (the dumbbell near your mid-section) and then lower the weight under control to the start/finish position (the dumbbell away from your mid-section) to ensure a sufficient stretch. After performing a set with your right arm, repeat the exercise for the other side of your body (while lying on your left side).

Training Tips:

• You shouldn't lie directly on your upper arm as you perform this exercise.

• Doing this exercise on a bench (instead of the floor) will increase your range of motion and permit a greater stretch.

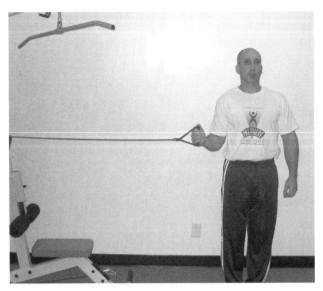
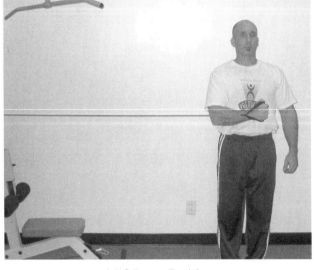

| *Start/Finish Position* | *Mid-Range Position* |

INTERNAL ROTATION (cable column)

Equipment Needed: cable column and handle

Muscles Influenced: internal rotators

Suggested Repetitions: 6 - 12

Start/Finish Position: Adjust the position of the pulley so that it's approximately even with your right elbow. Grasp the handle with your right hand and turn your feet so that your right side is facing the machine. Slide your feet away from the machine so that the weight you intend to lift is separated slightly from the rest of the weight stack. Position your left hand on your left hip (or allow your left arm to hang straight down). Place your right elbow against the right side of your torso and bend your right arm so that the angle between your upper and lower arms is about 90 degrees. (By doing this, your right lower arm will be approximately parallel to the floor.) Position the handle away from your mid-section and spread your feet about shoulder-width apart.

Performance Description: Without moving your elbow away from the side of your torso or changing the angle of your arm, pull the handle to your mid-section. Pause briefly in this mid-range position (the handle near your mid-section) and then return the weight under control to the start/finish position (the handle away from your mid-section) to ensure a sufficient stretch. After performing a set with your right arm, repeat the exercise for the other side of your body.

Training Tips:

• Keep your elbow against the side of your torso and your lower arm parallel to the floor as you perform this exercise.

• Don't rotate your torso as you perform this exercise – movement should only occur around your shoulder joint.

• You can also perform this exercise with a resistance band/cord. You'd secure the band/cord to an object that will not move at a height that's approximately even with your elbow. Otherwise, the exercise would be performed in the same fashion as described above.

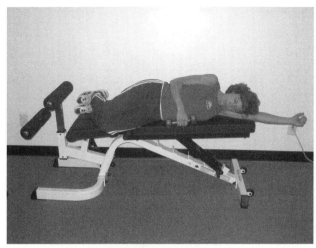
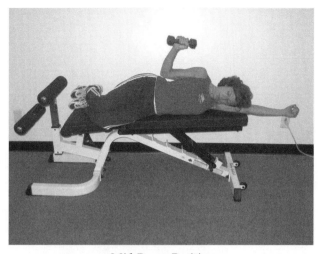

Start/Finish Position   *Mid-Range Position*

EXTERNAL ROTATION

Equipment Needed: dumbbell and bench

Muscles Influenced: external rotators

Suggested Repetitions: 6 - 12

Start/Finish Position: Grasp a dumbbell with your right hand, lie down on the back pad of a bench on your left side and draw your knees toward your torso. Position your left arm just in front of your torso and lean back slightly. Keep your right elbow against your side and bend your right arm so that the angle between your upper and lower arms is about 90 degrees. Point your right palm downward.

Performance Description: Without moving your elbow or changing the angle of your arm, raise the dumbbell as high as possible. Pause briefly in this mid-range position (the dumbbell away from your mid-section) and then lower the weight under control to the start/finish position (the dumbbell near your mid-section) to obtain a proper stretch. After performing a set with your right arm, repeat the exercise for the other side of your body (while lying on your right side).

Training Tips:

• Don't rotate your torso as you perform this exercise – movement should only occur around your shoulder joint.

• Doing this exercise on a bench (instead of the floor) will increase your range of motion and permit a greater stretch.

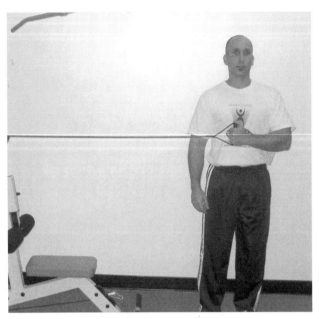

Start/Finish Position

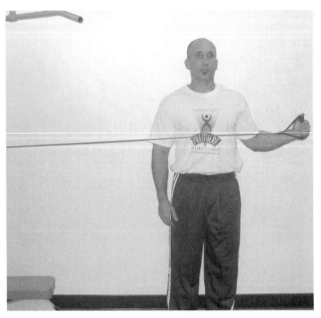

Mid-Range Position

EXTERNAL ROTATION (cable column)

Equipment Needed: cable column and handle

Muscles Influenced: external rotators

Suggested Repetitions: 6 - 12

Start/Finish Position: Adjust the position of the pulley so that it's approximately even with your left elbow. Grasp the handle with your left hand and turn your feet so that your right side is facing the machine. Slide your feet away from the machine so that the weight you intend to lift is separated slightly from the rest of the weight stack. Position your right hand on your right hip (or allow your right arm to hang straight down). Place your left elbow against the left side of your torso and bend your left arm so that the angle between your upper and lower arms is about 90 degrees. (By doing this, your left lower arm will be approximately parallel to the floor.) Position the handle against your mid-section and spread your feet about shoulder-width apart.

Performance Description: Without moving your elbow away from the side of your torso or changing the angle of your arm, pull the handle away from your mid-section. Pause briefly in this mid-range position (the handle away from your mid-section) and then return the weight under control to the start/finish position (the handle near your mid-section) to ensure a sufficient stretch. After performing a set with your left arm, repeat the exercise for the other side of your body.

Training Tips:

• Keep your elbow against the side of your torso and your lower arm parallel to the floor as you perform this exercise.

• Don't rotate your torso as you perform this exercise – movement should only occur around your shoulder joint.

• Your palm should be facing you in the start/finish position.

• You can also perform this exercise with a resistance band/cord. You'd secure the band/cord to an object that will not move at a height that's approximately even with your elbow. Otherwise, the exercise would be performed in the same fashion as described above.

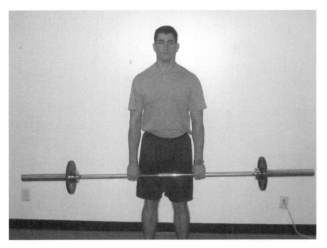

Start/Finish Position

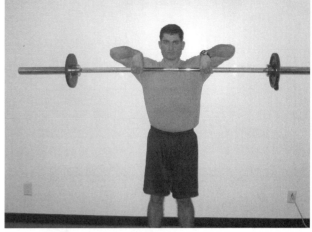

Mid-Range Position

UPRIGHT ROW

Equipment Needed: barbell or dumbbells

Muscles Influenced: trapezius (upper portion), biceps and forearms

Suggested Repetitions: 6 - 12

Start/Finish Position: Reach down and grasp a bar with your hands spaced slightly narrower than shoulder-width apart and your palms facing you. Stand upright by straightening your legs and torso. Straighten your arms and spread your feet about shoulder-width apart.

Performance Description: Pull the bar up until it's just below your chin. (Your elbows should be slightly higher than your hands in this position.) Pause briefly in this mid-range position (your arms flexed) and then return the bar under control to the start/finish position (your arms fully extended) to ensure a proper stretch.

Training Tips:

• Avoid throwing the weight by using your legs or swinging your torso back and forth – movement should only occur around your shoulder and elbow joints.

• You can also perform this exercise with dumbbells in the same fashion as described above.

• You can also perform this exercise with a cable column. You'd adjust the position of the pulley so that it's near the bottom of the column and attach a bar. In addition, you'd slide your feet away from the machine so that the weight you intend to lift is separated slightly from the rest of the weight stack. Otherwise, the exercise would be performed in the same fashion as described above.

• For better biomechanical leverage, you should keep the bar (or the dumbbells) close to your body as you perform this exercise.

• You can use wrist straps if you have difficulty in maintaining your grip on the bar (or the dumbbells).

• This exercise may be contraindicated if you have shoulder-impingement syndrome. In this case, however, raising the bar to the lower part of your chest (near the tip of your breastbone) rather than to the upper part of it will reduce the stress on an impinged shoulder. This exercise may also be contraindicated if you have low-back pain or hyperextended elbows.

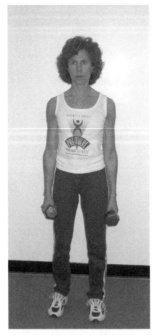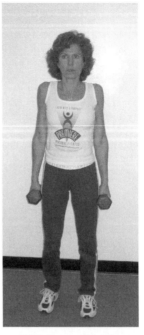

Start/Finish Position   *Mid-Range Position*

SHOULDER SHRUG

Equipment Needed: dumbbells, barbell or trap bar

Muscle Influenced: trapezius (upper portion)

Suggested Repetitions: 8 - 12

Start/Finish Position: Reach down and grasp a dumbbell in each hand on the outside of your legs with a "parallel grip" (your palms facing each other). Stand upright by straightening your legs and torso. Straighten your arms and spread your feet about shoulder-width apart.

Performance Description: Keep your arms and legs fairly straight and pull the dumbbells up as high as possible trying to touch your shoulders to your ears (as if to say, "I don't know"). Pause briefly in this mid-range position (your shoulders near your ears) and then lower the dumbbells under control to the start/finish position (your shoulders away from your ears) to obtain an adequate stretch.

Training Tips:

• It isn't necessary or advisable for you to "roll" your shoulders as you perform this exercise.

• Avoid throwing the weight by using your legs or swinging your torso back and forth – movement should only occur around your shoulder joints.

• You can also perform this exercise with a barbell and trap bar. When doing this exercise with a barbell, you should grasp the bar with both hands approximately shoulder-width apart with your palms facing you. Otherwise, the exercise would be performed in the same fashion as described above.

• For better biomechanical leverage, you should keep the dumbbells (or the bar) close to your body as you perform this exercise.

• You can use wrist straps if you have difficulty in maintaining your grip on the dumbbells (or the bar).

• This exercise may be contraindicated if you have low-back pain or hyperextended elbows.

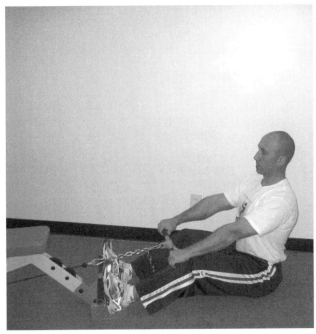

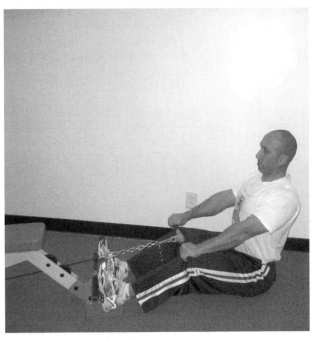

Start/Finish Position

Mid-Range Position

SCAPULA RETRACTION

Equipment Needed: cable column and bar

Muscles Influenced: trapezius (middle portion)

Suggested Repetitions: 8 - 12

Start/Finish Position: Adjust the position of the pulley so that it's near the bottom of the column and attach a bar. Sit down on the floor, grasp the bar with your palms facing down and space your hands approximately shoulder-width apart. Straighten your legs but maintain a slight bend at your knees and sit upright. Adjust the position of your legs so that the weight you intend to lift is separated slightly from the rest of the weight stack. Lean back slightly.

Performance Description: Keep your arms fairly straight and "pinch" your shoulder blades together. Pause briefly in this mid-range position (your shoulder blades together) and then lower the weight under control to the start/finish position (your shoulder blades apart) to ensure a sufficient stretch.

Training Tips:

- It's natural for you to change the position of your torso as you perform this exercise. However, movement of your torso shouldn't be excessive or used to throw the weight – movement should only occur around your shoulder joints.

- Don't slam the weights together between repetitions.

- You can do this exercise unilaterally (one limb at a time) if you have a shoulder or arm injury, a gross difference in the strength between your limbs or desire a training variation. (To do the exercise unilaterally requires a handle instead of a bar.)

- You can use wrist straps if you have difficulty in maintaining your grip on the bar.

- This exercise may be contraindicated if you have hyperextended elbows.

12

THE UPPER ARMS

Because your upper arms contain a relatively small amount of muscle mass, they're regarded as the "weak links" in multiple-joint movements for your torso. Therefore, it's critical for you to exercise these smaller, weaker muscles in order to strengthen the weak link.

MUSCLES OF THE UPPER ARMS

The two main muscles of your upper arms are the biceps and triceps.

Biceps

The prominent muscle that's located on the front of your upper arm is technically known as the "biceps brachii." As the name suggests, the biceps have two separate parts (or "heads"). The separation can sometimes be seen as a groove on a well-developed upper arm when the biceps are fully contracted. The primary function of your biceps is elbow flexion (bending your arms). Your biceps assist the muscles of your torso – especially your "lats" – in climbing skills and pulling movements.

Triceps

The prominent muscle that's located on the back of your upper arm is technically known as the "triceps brachii." As the name suggests, the triceps have three distinct heads: the long, lateral and medial. These three heads produce a horseshoe-shaped appearance on a well-developed upper arm when the triceps are fully contracted. The primary function of your triceps is elbow extension (straightening your arms). Your triceps assist the muscles of your torso in throwing skills and pushing movements.

EXERCISES FOR THE UPPER ARMS

This chapter will describe and illustrate eight exercises that you can perform for the muscles of your upper arm. The exercises are the bicep curl, preacher curl, concentration curl, bicep curl (with a cable column), tricep extension, tricep extension (with a cable column), French curl and tricep kickback.

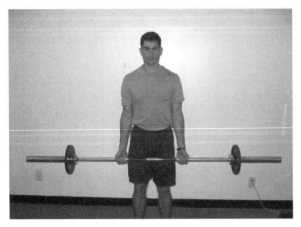
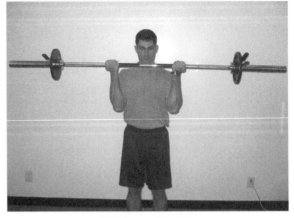

Start/Finish Position	Mid-Range Position

BICEP CURL

Equipment Needed: barbell, EZ-curl bar or dumbbells

Muscles Influenced: biceps and forearms

Suggested Repetitions: 6 - 12

Start/Finish Position: Reach down and grasp a bar with your hands spaced slightly wider than shoulder-width apart and your palms facing away from you. Stand upright by straightening your legs and torso. Straighten your arms and spread your feet approximately shoulder-width apart.

Performance Description: Keep your elbows against the sides of your torso and pull the bar below your chin by bending your arms. Pause briefly in this mid-range position (your arms flexed) and then lower the weight under control to the start/finish position (your arms fully extended) to provide a sufficient stretch.

Training Tips:

- Avoid throwing the weight by using your legs or swinging your torso back and forth – movement should only occur around your elbow joints.

- It's natural for you to change the position of your upper arms as you perform this exercise. However, movement of your upper arms shouldn't be excessive.

- You can also perform this exercise with an EZ-curl bar and dumbbells in a similar fashion as described above.

- You can also perform this exercise with a cable column. You'd adjust the position of the pulley so that it's near the bottom of the column and attach a bar. In addition, you'd slide your feet away from the machine so that the weight you intend to lift is separated slightly from the rest of the weight stack. Otherwise, the exercise would be performed in the same fashion as described above.

- You can do this exercise unilaterally (one limb at a time) if you have an arm injury, a gross difference in the strength between your limbs or desire a training variation. (To do the exercise unilaterally requires a dumbbell instead of a barbell or, with a cable column, a handle instead of a bar.)

- This exercise may be contraindicated if you have hyperextended elbows.

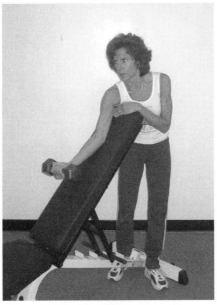
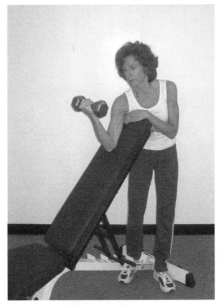

Start/Finish Position   *Mid-Range Position*

PREACHER CURL

Equipment Needed: dumbbell and adjustable bench

Muscles Influenced: biceps and forearms

Suggested Repetitions: 6 - 12

Start/Finish Position: Adjust the position of the bench so that the back pad is inclined at about a 45-degree angle. Reach down and grasp a dumbbell with your right hand. Stand upright by straightening your legs and torso. Step behind the bench and place the back of your right upper arm on the pad. Straighten your right arm and position your right hand so that your palm is facing upward.

Performance Description: Keep your upper arm against the pad and pull the dumbbell below your chin by bending your arm. Pause briefly in this mid-range position (your arm flexed) and then lower the weight under control to the start/finish position (your arm fully extended) to provide a sufficient stretch. Repeat the exercise for the other side of your body.

Training Tips:

- Avoid throwing the weight by using your legs or swinging your torso back and forth – movement should only occur around your elbow joint.

- You can also perform this exercise with a cable column. You'd adjust the position of the pulley so that it's near the bottom of the column and attach a handle. In addition, you'd position the bench away from the machine so that the weight you intend to lift is separated slightly from the rest of the weight stack. Otherwise, the exercise would be performed in the same fashion as described above.

- This exercise may be contraindicated if you have a hyperextended elbow.

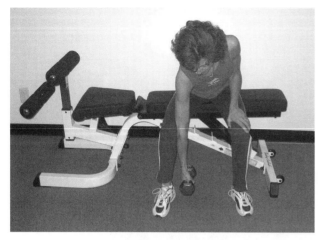
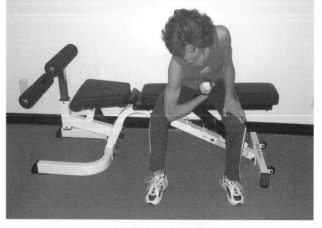

| *Start/Finish Position* | *Mid-Range Position* |

CONCENTRATION CURL

Equipment Needed: dumbbell and bench (or chair or stool)

Muscles Influenced: biceps and forearm

Suggested Repetitions: 6 - 12

Start/Finish Position: Reach down and grasp a dumbbell with your right hand. Sit down near the end of the back pad of a bench and place your feet flat on the floor. Place the back of your right upper arm against the inside of your right upper leg. Straighten your right arm and position your hand so that your palm is facing away from your right leg. Place your left lower arm on top of your left upper leg.

Performance Description: Keep your upper arm against the inside of your upper leg and pull the dumbbell below your chin by bending your arm. Pause briefly in this mid-range position (your arm flexed) and then lower the weight under control to the start/finish position (your arm fully extended) to provide a sufficient stretch. After performing a set with your right arm, repeat the exercise for the other side of your body.

Training Tips:

• Avoid throwing the weight by using your legs or swinging your torso back and forth – movement should only occur around your elbow joint.

• You can also perform this exercise with a cable column. You'd adjust the position of the pulley so that it's near the bottom of the column and attach a handle. In addition, you'd position the bench away from the machine so that the weight you intend to lift is separated slightly from the rest of the weight stack. Otherwise, the exercise would be performed in the same fashion as described above.

• This exercise may be contraindicated if you have a hyperextended elbow.

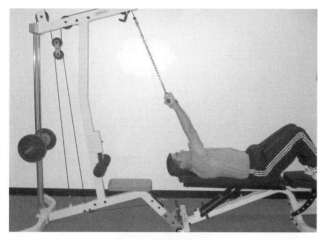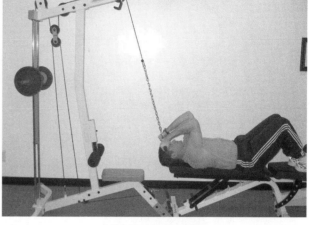

| Start/Finish Position | Mid-Range Position |

BICEP CURL (cable column)

Equipment Needed: cable column, bar and bench

Muscles Influenced: biceps and forearms

Suggested Repetitions: 6 - 12

Start/Finish Position: Adjust the position of the pulley so that it's near the top of the column and attach a bar. Reach up and grasp the bar with your hands spaced slightly wider than shoulder-width apart and your palms facing toward you. Sit down near the end of the back pad of a bench and place your feet flat on the floor. Lie down on the pad and position your upper arms so that they're approximately perpendicular to the floor.

Performance Description: Keep your upper arms approximately perpendicular to the floor and pull the bar near your forehead by bending your arms. Pause briefly in this mid-range position (your arms flexed) and then lower the weight under control to the start/finish position (your arms fully extended) to provide a sufficient stretch.

Training Tips:

• Keep your torso against the pad and your feet flat on the floor as you perform this exercise. If you have low-back pain, you can place your feet on the end of the pad, a chair or a stool. This will flatten your lumbar area against the pad and reduce the stress in your low-back region.

• It's natural for you to change the position of your upper arms as you perform this exercise. However, movement of your upper arms shouldn't be excessive.

• You can do this exercise unilaterally (one limb at a time) if you have an arm injury, a gross difference in the strength between your limbs or desire a training variation. (To do the exercise unilaterally requires a handle instead of a bar.)

• This exercise may be contraindicated if you have shoulder-impingement syndrome or hyperextended elbows.

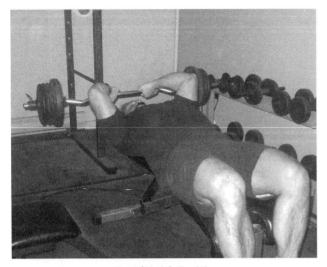
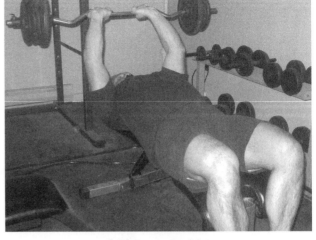

Start/Finish Position   *Mid-Range Position*

TRICEP EXTENSION

Equipment Needed: EZ-curl bar, barbell or dumbbells and bench

Muscle Influenced: triceps

Suggested Repetitions: 6 - 12

Start/Finish Position: Reach down and grasp an EZ-curl bar with your palms facing you. Sit down near the end of the back pad of a bench and place your feet flat on the floor. Lie down on the pad, raise the bar above your chest and straighten your arms. Position your upper arms so that they're approximately perpendicular to the floor, spread your hands about 4 - 6 inches apart and point your elbows toward your knees. (Another person may be needed to position a heavy weight.) Lower the bar until it's near your forehead by bending your arms. (How close the bar is to your forehead depends upon the length of your lower arms).

Performance Description: Keep your upper arms approximately perpendicular to the floor and your elbows pointing toward your knees and push the bar up by straightening your arms. Pause briefly in this mid-range position (your arms extended) and then return the weight under control to the start/finish position (your arms flexed) to obtain a proper stretch.

Training Tips:

• Keep your torso against the pad and your feet flat on the floor as you perform this exercise. If you have low-back pain, you can place your feet on the end of the pad or a chair or stool. This will flatten your lumbar area against the pad and reduce the stress in your low-back region.

• It's natural for you to change the position of your upper arms as you perform this exercise. However, movement of your upper arms shouldn't be excessive.

• You can also perform this exercise with a barbell and dumbbells in a similar fashion as described above. (When using dumbbells, your hands should face each other.)

• You can do this exercise unilaterally (one limb at a time) if you have an arm injury, a gross difference in the strength between your limbs or desire a training variation. (To do the exercise unilaterally requires a dumbbell instead of an EZ-curl bar.)

• This exercise may be contraindicated if you have shoulder-impingement syndrome.

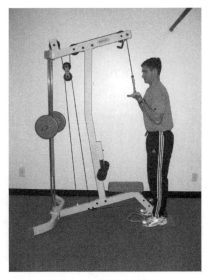 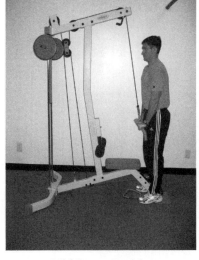

Start/Finish Position   *Mid-Range Position*

TRICEP EXTENSION (cable column)

Equipment Needed: cable column and bar

Muscle Influenced: triceps

Suggested Repetitions: 6 - 12

Start/Finish Position: Adjust the position of the pulley so that it's near the top of the column and attach a bar. Reach up and grasp the bar with your hands spaced about 4 - 6 inches apart and your palms facing downward. Take a step or two backward and spread your feet approximately shoulder-width apart (or place one foot slightly in front of the other). Pull the bar down until your upper arms are against the sides of your torso.

Performance Description: Keep your upper arms against the sides of your torso and push the bar down by straightening your arms. Pause briefly in this mid-range position (your arms fully extended) and then return the weight under control to the start/finish position (your arms flexed) to ensure a proper stretch.

Training Tips:

- Your upper arms should remain in contact with the sides of your torso as you perform this exercise.

- Avoid swinging your torso back and forth as you perform this exercise – movement should only occur around your elbow joints.

- You can do this exercise unilaterally (one limb at a time) if you have an arm injury, a gross difference in the strength between your limbs or desire a training variation. (To do the exercise unilaterally requires a handle instead of a bar.)

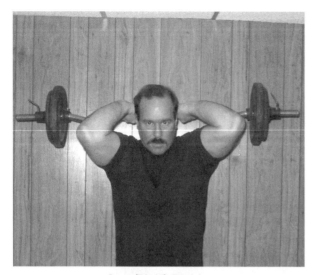

Start/Finish Position

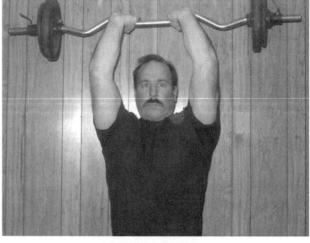

Mid-Range Position

FRENCH CURL

Equipment Needed: EZ-curl bar or dumbbell

Muscle Influenced: triceps

Suggested Repetitions: 6 - 12

Start/Finish Position: Reach down and grasp an EZ-curl bar with your hands spaced about 4 - 6 inches apart and your palms facing you. Stand upright by straightening your legs and torso. Raise the bar above your head and straighten your arms. Position your upper arms so that they're approximately perpendicular to the floor and point your elbows forward. (Another person may be needed to position a heavy weight.) Lower the bar behind your head until it's near the base of your neck by bending your arms and spread your feet approximately shoulder-width apart.

Performance Description: Keep your upper arms approximately perpendicular to the floor and push the bar up by straightening your arms. Pause briefly in this mid-range position (your arms extended) and then return the weight under control to the start/finish position (your arms flexed) to obtain a proper stretch.

Training Tips:

• Avoid swinging your torso back and forth as you perform this exercise – movement should only occur around your elbow joints.

• It's natural for you to change the position of your upper arms as you perform this exercise. However, movement of your upper arms shouldn't be excessive.

• You can do this exercise unilaterally (one limb at a time) if you have an arm injury, a gross difference in the strength between your limbs or desire a training variation. (To do the exercise unilaterally requires a dumbbell instead of a bar.)

• This exercise may be contraindicated if you have shoulder-impingement syndrome.

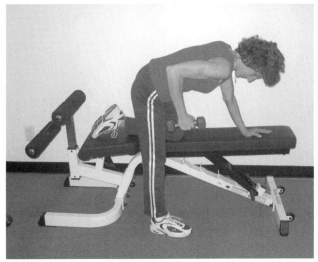
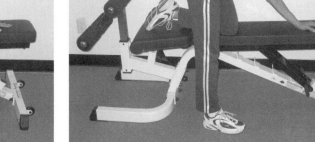

| Start/Finish Position | Mid-Range Position |

TRICEP KICKBACK

Equipment Needed: dumbbell and bench

Muscle Influenced: triceps

Suggested Repetitions: 6 - 12

Start/Finish Position: Place your left hand and left knee on the back pad of a bench. Position your right foot on the floor at a comfortable distance from the bench. Reach down and grasp a dumbbell with your right hand. Position your right upper arm against the right side of your torso and allow your right lower arm to hang straight down. Your right palm should be facing the bench.

Performance Description: Keep your upper arm against the side of your torso and push the weight up by straightening your arm. Pause briefly in this mid-range position (your arm extended) and then return the weight under control to the start/finish position (your arm flexed) to obtain a proper stretch. After performing a set with your right arm, repeat the exercise for the other side of your body (with your right hand and right knee on the back pad for support).

Training Tips:

• It's natural for you to change the position of your upper arm as you perform this exercise. However, movement of your upper arm shouldn't be excessive or used to throw the dumbbell – movement should only occur around your elbow joint.

13

THE LOWER ARMS

Your lower arms contain a relatively small amount of muscle mass and are regarded as the "weak links" in multiple-joint movements for the torso. Therefore, it's critical for you to exercise these smaller, weaker muscles in order to strengthen the weak link.

MUSCLES OF THE LOWER ARMS

The forearms are the major muscles in your lower arms.

Forearms

Amazingly as it may seem, each one of your forearms is made up of 19 different muscles. These muscles may be divided into two groups on the basis of their position and function. The anterior group on the front of your forearm causes wrist flexion (flexing your wrist) and pronation (turning your palm downward); the posterior group on the back of your forearm causes wrist extension (extending your wrist) and supination (turning your palm upward). Since the muscles of your forearms affect your wrists, hands and fingers, they're extremely important in pulling movements, climbing skills and tasks that involve gripping.

EXERCISES FOR THE LOWER ARMS

This chapter will describe and illustrate four exercises that you can perform for the muscles of your lower arms. The exercises are wrist flexion, wrist extension, wrist roller and finger flexion.

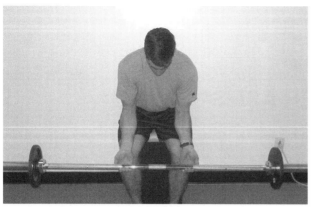

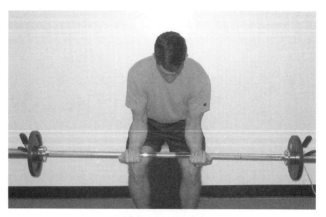

Start/Finish Position   *Mid-Range Position*

WRIST FLEXION

Equipment Needed: barbell or dumbbells and bench (or chair or stool)

Muscles Influenced: wrist flexors

Suggested Repetitions: 8 - 12

Start/Finish Position: Reach down and grasp a bar with your palms facing away from you. Lift the bar, sit down near the end of the back pad of a bench (or a chair or stool) and place the backs of your forearms directly over your upper legs. (You can also place your forearms flat on the pad between your legs.) Place your thumbs underneath the bar alongside your fingers and spread your hands about 4 - 6 inches apart. Lean forward slightly so that the angle between your upper and lower arms is about 90 degrees or less. Your wrists should be over your kneecaps (or over the edge of the pad if you placed your forearms on it).

Performance Description: Pull the bar up as high as possible by flexing your wrists. Pause briefly in this mid-range position (your wrists flexed) and then lower the weight under control to the start/finish position (your wrists extended) to provide a sufficient stretch.

Training Tips:

• Your forearms should remain directly over your upper legs throughout the performance of this exercise.

• Placing your thumbs underneath the bar alongside your fingers will give you a greater range of motion.

• Avoid throwing the weight by using your legs or swinging your torso back and forth – movement should only occur around your wrist joints.

• You can also perform this exercise with dumbbells in a similar fashion as described above.

• You can also perform this exercise with a cable column. You'd adjust the position of the pulley so that it's near the bottom of the column and attach a bar. In addition, you'd slide the bench away from the machine so that the weight you intend to lift is separated slightly from the rest of the weight stack. Otherwise, the exercise would be performed in the same fashion as described above.

• You can do this exercise unilaterally (one limb at a time) if you have an arm injury, a gross difference in the strength between your limbs or desire a training variation. (To do the exercise unilaterally requires a dumbbell instead of a barbell.)

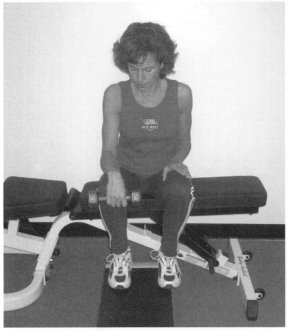

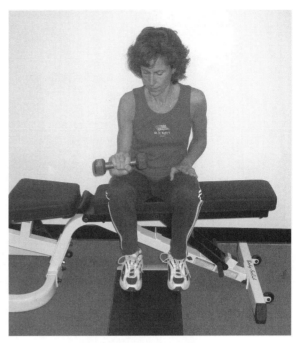

Start/Finish Position   *Mid-Range Position*

WRIST EXTENSION

Equipment Needed: dumbbell and bench (or chair or stool)

Muscles Influenced: wrist extensors

Suggested Repetitions: 8 - 12

Start/Finish Position: Reach down and grasp a dumbbell with your right hand. Lift the dumbbell, sit down near the end of the back pad of a bench (or a chair or stool) and place the front of your right forearm directly over your right upper leg so that your palm is facing down. (You can also place your right forearm flat on the pad between your legs.) Lean forward slightly so that the angle between your upper and lower arms is about 90 degrees or less. Your right wrist should be over your right kneecap (or over the edge of the pad if you placed your forearm on it).

Performance Description: Pull the dumbbell up as high as possible by extending your wrist. Pause briefly in this mid-range position (your wrist extended) and then lower the weight under control to the start/finish position (your wrist flexed) to obtain an adequate stretch. After performing a set with your right arm, repeat the exercise for the other side of your body.

Training Tips:

• Your forearm should remain directly over your upper leg throughout the performance of this exercise.

• Avoid throwing the weight by using your leg or swinging your torso back and forth – movement should only occur around your wrist joint.

• This exercise is more comfortable on your wrist when it's performed one limb at a time with a dumbbell rather than both limbs at a time with a barbell.

• You can also perform this exercise with a cable column. You'd adjust the position of the pulley so that it's near the bottom of the column and attach a handle. In addition, you'd slide the bench away from the machine so that the weight you intend to lift is separated slightly from the rest of the weight stack. Otherwise, the exercise would be performed in the same fashion as described above.

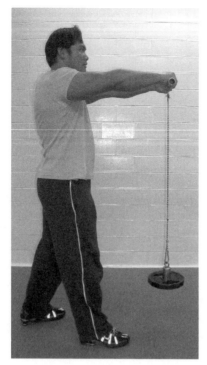 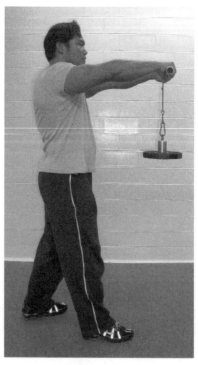

Start/Finish Position   *Mid-Range Position*

WRIST ROLLER

Equipment Needed: roller bar

Muscles Influenced: wrist flexors, wrist extensors and anterior deltoids

Suggested Repetitions: 1 - 2 (or 50 - 70 seconds)

Start/Finish Position: Reach down and grasp a roller bar with your palms facing you. Stand upright by straightening your legs and torso. Raise your arms forward until they're parallel to the floor. Straighten your arms and spread your feet a comfortable distance apart with one foot slightly in front of the other.

Performance Description: Keep your arms fairly straight and parallel to the floor and alternately extend your wrists until the rope is completely wound around the bar. (In other words, extend your right wrist while allowing the bar to "roll" freely in your left hand then extend your left wrist while allowing the bar to "roll" freely in your right hand.) Return the weight under control to the start/finish position by alternately flexing your wrists until the rope is completely unwound.

Training Tips:

- Avoid throwing the weight by using your legs or swinging your torso back and forth – movement should only occur around your wrist joints.

- You can do this exercise for a prescribed number of repetitions or a designated amount of time. (Note: One repetition counts as completely winding the rope around the bar and then unwinding it.)

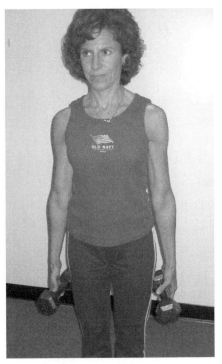
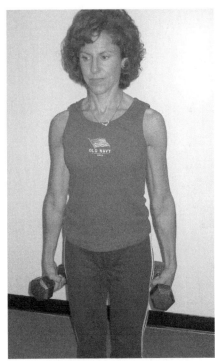

Start/Finish Position   *Mid-Range Position*

FINGER FLEXION

Equipment Needed: dumbbells or barbell

Muscles Influenced: finger flexors

Suggested Repetitions: 8 - 12

Start/Finish Position: Reach down and grasp a dumbbell in each hand. Stand upright by straightening your legs and torso. Hold the dumbbells at the sides of your body with your palms facing your legs and spread your feet about shoulder-width apart. Straighten your arms and allow the dumbbells to roll down your hands to your fingertips.

Performance Description: Keep your arms fairly straight and pull the dumbbells up to your thumbs. Pause briefly in this mid-range position (your fingers flexed) and then lower the dumbbells under control to the start/finish position (your fingers extended) to ensure an adequate stretch.

Training Tips:

- Avoid throwing the dumbbells by using your legs or arms – movement should only occur around your finger joints.
- Squeeze the dumbbells as hard as possible in the mid-range position.
- Attempt to lower the dumbbells all the way down to your fingertips – to the point where the dumbbells almost drop from your fingers.
- You can also perform this exercise with a barbell. You'd keep the bar in front of your upper legs and grasp it either with your palms facing you or away from you. Otherwise, the exercise would be performed in the same fashion as described above.
- You can also perform this exercise with a cable column. You'd adjust the position of the pulley so that it's near the bottom of the column and attach a bar. Otherwise, the exercise would be performed in the same fashion as described above.
- You can do this exercise unilaterally (one limb at a time) if you have an arm injury, a gross difference in the strength between your limbs or desire a training variation.

14

THE ABDOMINALS

The muscles of the abdominals serve as an important link between your lower body and torso.

MUSCLES OF THE ABDOMINALS

The abdominal muscles are located on the anterior portion of your mid-section and are comprised of the rectus abdominis, obliques and transversus abdominis. These muscles perform a variety of functions.

Rectus Abdominis

This long, narrow muscle extends vertically across the front of your abdomen from the lower rim of your rib cage to your pelvis. Its main function is torso flexion (pulling your torso toward your lower body). The fibers of this muscle are interrupted along their course by three horizontal fibrous bands which gives rise to the term "washboard abs" when describing an especially well-developed abdomen. The rectus abdominis helps to control your breathing and plays a major role in forced expiration during intense exercise.

Obliques

The external and internal obliques reside on both sides of your mid-section. The external oblique is a broad muscle whose fibers form a V across the front of your abdominal area, extending diagonally downward from your lower ribs to your pubic bone. The external oblique has two main functions: torso lateral flexion (bending your torso to the same side) and torso rotation (turning your torso to the opposite side). The internal oblique is located immediately under the external oblique on both sides of your abdomen. The fibers of the internal oblique form an inverted V along the front of your abdominal wall, extending diagonally upward from your pubic bone to your ribs. The internal oblique has two main functions: torso lateral flexion (bending your torso to the same side) and torso rotation (turning your torso to the same side). In short, your external and internal obliques are used during movements in which your torso bends laterally or twists. These muscles are also active during expiration and inspiration, respectively.

Transversus Abdominis

The innermost layer of your abdominal musculature is the transversus abdominis. The fibers of this muscle run horizontally across your abdomen. The primary function of the transversus abdominis is to constrict your abdomen. This muscle is also involved in forced expiration and helps to control your breathing.

EXERCISES FOR THE ABDOMINALS

This chapter will describe and illustrate seven exercises that you can perform for the muscles of your abdominals. The exercises are the crunch, crunch (with a stability ball), crunch (with a cable column), knee-up, side bend, side bend (with a cable column) and rotary crunch.

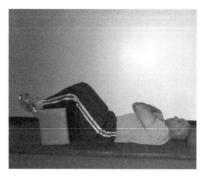
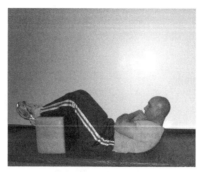

Start/Finish Position   Mid-Range Position

CRUNCH

Equipment Needed: bench, chair or stool

Muscles Influenced: rectus abdominis and iliopsoas

Suggested Repetitions: 10 - 12

Start/Finish Position: Lie down on the floor and place the backs of your lower legs on the back pad of a bench (or a chair or stool). Position yourself so that your upper legs are approximately perpendicular to the floor and the angle between your upper and lower legs is about 90 degrees. Fold your arms across your chest and lift your head off the floor. (The upper portion of your shoulder blades shouldn't touch the floor.)

Performance Description: Pull your torso as close to your upper legs as possible. Pause briefly in this mid-range position (your torso flexed) and then lower your torso under control to the start/finish position (your torso extended) to obtain a proper stretch.

Training Tips:

- Avoid throwing your torso forward or snapping your head forward as you perform this exercise – movement should only occur around your hip joint and mid-section.

- Your abdominals are used primarily during the first 30 degrees or so of this exercise. (Thereafter, your hip flexors accept most of the workload.) So, it isn't necessary to bring your torso all the way to your upper legs.

- You shouldn't contact the floor with the upper portion of your shoulder blades between repetitions. This removes the load from the target muscles.

- If a bench, chair or stool isn't available, you can do the exercise by placing your feet flat on the floor and positioning yourself so that the angle between your upper and lower legs is about 90 degrees. Here, you'd bring your torso toward your upper legs but stop short of the point where it's perpendicular to the floor. Otherwise, the exercise would be performed in the same fashion as described above.

- If you can do 12 repetitions or more with strict form using your bodyweight, you can increase the workload on your muscles by holding a weight across your chest or performing the exercise with a slower speed of movement.

- This exercise may be contraindicated if you have low-back pain.

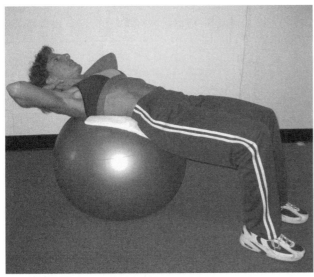
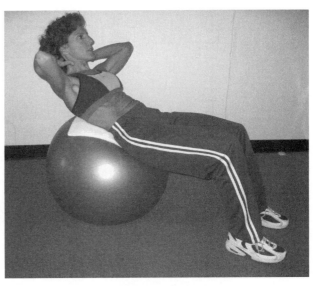

Start/Finish Position   *Mid-Range Position*

CRUNCH (ball)

Equipment Needed: stability ball

Muscles Influenced: rectus abdominis and iliopsoas

Suggested Repetitions: 10 - 12

Start/Finish Position: Lie down on a stability ball so that it's under your lower back. Position yourself so that the angle between your upper and lower legs is about 90 degrees. Place your feet flat on the floor and spread them apart a comfortable distance. Position your hands behind your head.

Performance Description: Pull your torso toward your upper legs. Pause briefly in this mid-range position (your torso flexed) and then lower your torso under control to the start/finish position (your torso extended) to obtain a proper stretch.

Training Tips:

- Avoid throwing your torso forward or snapping your head forward as you perform this exercise – movement should only occur around your hip joint and mid-section.

- Your abdominals are used primarily during the first 30 degrees or so of this exercise. (Thereafter, your hip flexors accept most of the workload.) So, it isn't necessary to bring your torso all the way to your upper legs. In fact, you should stop short of the point where it's perpendicular to the floor.

- If you can do 12 repetitions or more with strict form using your bodyweight, you can increase the workload on your muscles by holding a weight across your chest or performing the exercise with a slower speed of movement.

- This exercise may be contraindicated if you have low-back pain.

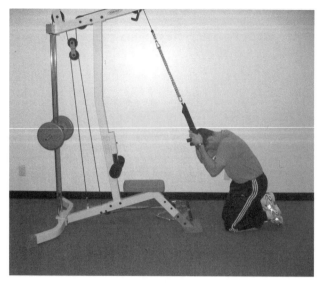

Start/Finish Position

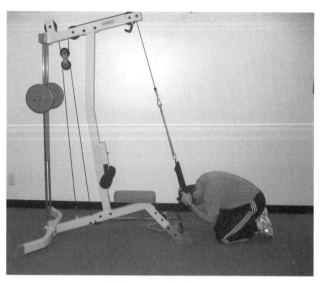

Mid-Range Position

CRUNCH (cable column)

Equipment Needed: cable column and rope handle

Muscles Influenced: rectus abdominis and iliopsoas

Suggested Repetitions: 10 - 12

Start/Finish Position: Adjust the position of the pulley so that it's near the top of the cable column and attach a rope handle. Reach up, grasp the rope and kneel on the floor. Pull the rope down so that your lower arms are against the sides of your head. Bend forward at the waist so that the angle between your torso and the floor is about 45 degrees.

Performance Description: Pull your torso toward your upper legs. Pause briefly in this mid-range position (your torso flexed) and then return your torso under control to the start/finish position (your torso extended) to obtain a proper stretch.

Training Tips:

• Avoid throwing your torso down or snapping your head down as you perform this exercise – movement should only occur around your hip joint and mid-section.

• This exercise may be contraindicated if you have low-back pain.

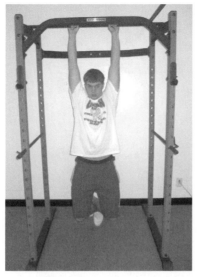
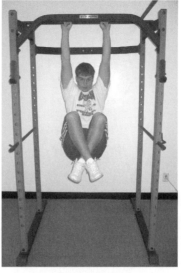

Start/Finish Position   *Mid-Range Position*

KNEE-UP

Equipment Needed: chin/pull-up bar or dip bars/handles

Muscles Influenced: iliopsoas and rectus abdominis (lower portion)

Suggested Repetitions: 8 - 12

Start/Finish Position: Reach up, grasp the bar with your palms facing away from you and space your hands several inches wider than shoulder-width apart. Bring your body to a "dead hang" and cross your ankles.

Performance Description: Pull your knees as close to your chest as possible. Pause briefly in this mid-range position (your knees near your chest) and then lower your legs under control to the start/finish position (your legs hanging down) to ensure a proper stretch.

Training Tips:

- Avoid swinging your body back and forth as you perform this exercise – movement should only occur around your hip and knee joints.

- If you use dip bars/handles for this exercise, you'd grasp the bars/handles and support your bodyweight by straightening your arms. Otherwise, the exercise would be performed in the same fashion as described above.

- If you can do 12 repetitions or more with strict form using your bodyweight, you can increase the workload on your muscles by performing the exercise with a slower speed of movement.

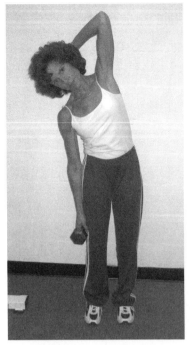
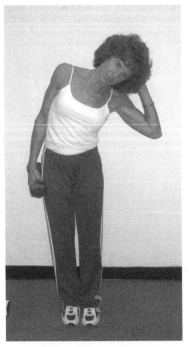

Start/Finish Position   *Mid-Range Position*

SIDE BEND

Equipment Needed: dumbbell

Muscles Influenced: obliques and erector spinae (lower back)

Suggested Repetitions: 10 - 12

Start/Finish Position: Reach down and grasp a dumbbell in your right hand. Stand upright by straightening your legs and torso. Hold the dumbbell against the right side of your body with your palm facing your leg and spread your feet about shoulder-width apart. Place your left palm against the left side of your head. Without moving your hips, bend your torso to the right as far as possible.

Performance Description: Without moving your hips, bring your torso to the left as far as possible. Pause briefly in this mid-range position (your torso bent to the left) and then lower the dumbbell under control to the start/finish position (your torso bent to the right) to ensure a sufficient stretch. After performing a set for the left side of your body, repeat the exercise for the other side of your body (holding the dumbbell in your left hand).

Training Tips:

• It's natural for you to change the position of your hips as you perform this exercise. However, movement of your hips shouldn't be excessive or used to throw the dumbbell – movement should only occur around your mid-section.

• Don't bend forward at the waist as you perform this exercise.

• Keep your feet flat on the floor as you perform this exercise.

• This exercise may be contraindicated if you have low-back pain.

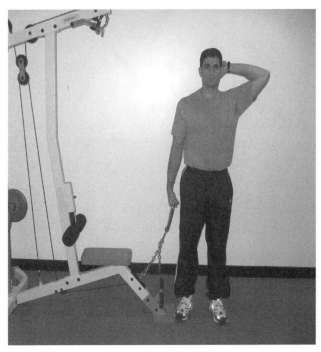
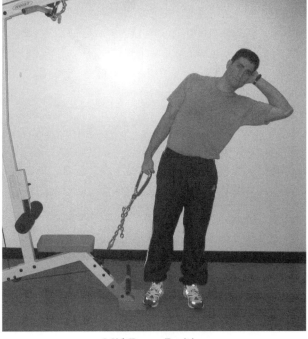

Start/Finish Position   *Mid-Range Position*

SIDE BEND (cable column)

Equipment Needed: cable column and handle

Muscles Influenced: obliques and erector spinae (lower back)

Suggested Repetitions: 10 - 12

Start/Finish Position: Adjust the position of the pulley so that it's near the floor and attach a handle. Reach down and grasp the handle with your right hand. Stand upright by straightening your legs and torso. Turn your feet to the left so that the right side of your body is facing the pulley. Slide your feet away from the machine so that the weight you intend to lift is separated slightly from the rest of the weight stack. Hold the handle near the right side of your body with your palm facing your leg and spread your feet about shoulder-width apart. Place your left palm against the left side of your head. Without moving your hips, bend your torso to the right as far as possible.

Performance Description: Without moving your hips, bring your torso to the left as far as possible. Pause briefly in this mid-range position (your torso bent to the left) and then lower the weight under control to the start/finish position (your torso bent to the right) to ensure a sufficient stretch. After performing a set for the left side of your body, repeat the exercise for the other side of your body (holding the handle with your left hand).

Training Tips:

• It's natural for you to change the position of your hips as you perform this exercise. However, movement of your hips shouldn't be excessive or used to throw the weight – movement should only occur around your mid-section.

• Don't bend forward at the waist as you perform this exercise.

• Keep your feet flat on the floor as you perform this exercise.

• This exercise may be contraindicated if you have low-back pain.

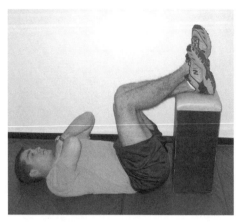
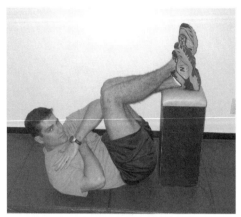

Start/Finish Position   *Mid-Range Position*

ROTARY CRUNCH

Equipment Needed: none

Muscles Involved: obliques and erector spinae (lower back)

Suggested Repetitions: 10 - 12

Start/Finish Position: Lie down on the floor and place the backs of your lower legs on top of a bench, chair or stool. Position yourself so that your upper legs are approximately perpendicular to the floor and the angle between your upper and lower legs is about 90 degrees. Fold your arms across your chest and lift your head off the floor. (The upper portion of your shoulder blades shouldn't touch the floor.)

Performance Description: Rotate your torso to the right as much as possible. Pause briefly in this mid-range position (your torso turned to the right) and then lower your torso under control to the start/finish position (your torso extended) to obtain a proper stretch. After performing a set for the right side of your body, repeat the exercise for the other side of your body (rotating your torso to the left).

Training Tips:

• Avoid throwing your torso forward or snapping your head forward as you perform this exercise – movement should only occur around your hip joint and mid-section.

• Your head should rotate in unison with your torso as you perform this exercise.

• You shouldn't contact the floor with the upper portion of your shoulder blades between repetitions. This removes the load from the target muscles.

• If a bench, chair or stool isn't available, you can do the exercise by placing your feet flat on the floor and positioning yourself so that the angle between your upper and lower legs is about 90 degrees. Here, you'd rotate your torso toward your upper legs but stop short of the point where it's perpendicular to the floor. Otherwise, the exercise would be performed in the same fashion as described above.

• If you can do 12 repetitions or more with strict form using your bodyweight, you can increase the workload on your muscles by holding a weight across your chest or performing the exercise with a slower speed of movement.

• This exercise may be contraindicated if you have low-back pain.

15

THE LOWER BACK

The muscles of your lower back serve as an important link between your lower body and torso.

MUSCLES OF THE LOWER BACK

The lower back muscles are located on the posterior portion of your mid-section. Today, low-back pain remains one of the most common and costly medical problems. It has been estimated that 80% of the world's population will experience low-back pain sometime in their lives with annual costs of more than $50 billion. Insufficient strength seems to be a factor related to low-back pain.

Erector Spinae

The main muscles in your lower back are the erector spinae (or "spinal erectors"). Their primary purpose is torso extension (straightening your torso from a bent-over position). However, the erector spinae also assist in torso lateral flexion (bending your torso to the side) and torso rotation (turning your torso).

EXERCISES FOR THE LOWER BACK

This chapter will describe and illustrate three exercises that you can perform for the muscles of your lower back. The exercises are the stiff-leg deadlift, back extension and back extension (with a stability ball).

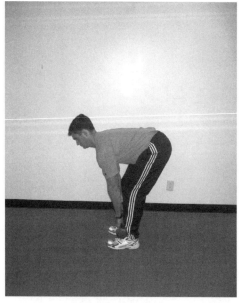
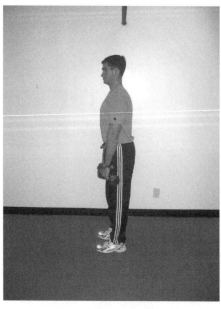

Start/Finish Position | *Mid-Range Position*

STIFF-LEG DEADLIFT

Equipment Needed: dumbbells, barbell or trap bar

Muscles Influenced: erector spinae (lower back), gluteus maximus (buttocks) and hamstrings

Suggested Repetitions: 10 - 15

Start/Finish Position: Spread your feet slightly narrower than shoulder-width apart. Reach down and grasp a dumbbell in each hand in front of your legs with your palms facing your body. Straighten your legs – but don't "lock" them – and your arms. Place most of your bodyweight on your heels, not on the balls of your feet.

Performance Description: Stand upright by straightening your torso. Pause briefly in this mid-range position (your torso extended) and then lower the weight under control to the start/finish position (your torso flexed) to ensure an adequate stretch.

Training Tips:

• Keep your arms and legs straight as you perform this exercise. Unlike the deadlift (described in Chapter 6), you should do most of the work with your lower back with little assistance from your hips and legs.

• You should exert force through your heels, not the balls of your feet.

• You shouldn't "lock" or "snap" your knees in the mid-range position of a repetition. This removes the load from the target muscles and may hyperextend your knees.

• You can also perform this exercise with a barbell and trap bar. When doing this exercise with a barbell, you should use an "alternating grip" (your dominant palm forward and non-dominant palm backward); when doing this exercise with a trap bar, you should use a "parallel" grip (your palms facing each other). Otherwise, the exercise would be performed in the same fashion as described above.

• When using a barbell or trap bar, don't bounce the weight off the floor between repetitions.

• You can use wrist straps if you have difficulty in maintaining your grip on the dumbbells (or the bar).

• This exercise may be contraindicated if you have low-back pain, hyperextended elbows or an exceptionally long torso and/or legs.

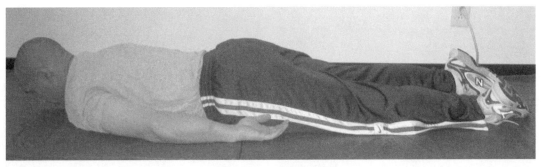

Start/Finish Position

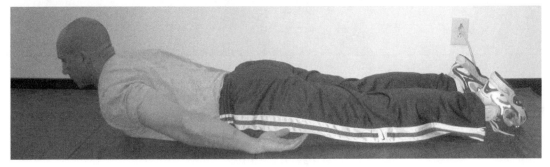

Mid-Range Position

BACK EXTENSION

Equipment Needed: none

Muscles Influenced: erector spinae (lower back) and gluteus maximus (buttocks)

Suggested Repetitions: 10 - 15

Start/Finish Position: Lie prone on the floor and place your arms at your sides. Straighten your legs and bring them together. Look straight ahead.

Performance Description: Raise your torso as high as possible. Pause briefly in this mid-range position (your torso extended) and then lower your torso under control to the start/finish position (your torso flexed) to obtain a sufficient stretch.

Training Tips:

- Avoid throwing your torso backward or snapping your head backward as you perform this exercise – movement should only occur around your hip joint and mid-section.

- If you can do 15 repetitions or more with strict form using your bodyweight, you can increase the workload on your muscles by performing the exercise with a slower speed of movement.

- This exercise may be contraindicated if you have low-back pain.

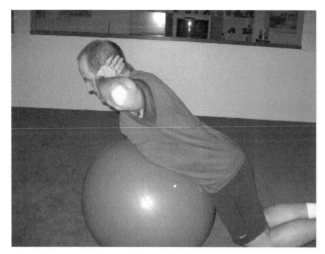
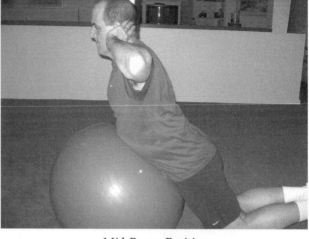

Start/Finish Position   *Mid-Range Position*

BACK EXTENSION (ball)

Equipment Needed: stability ball

Muscles Influenced: erector spinae (lower back) and gluteus maximus (buttocks)

Suggested Repetitions: 10 - 15

Start/Finish Position: Kneel down on the floor and position your torso on a stability ball so that it's under your mid-section. Place your hands against the sides of your head and bend forward.

Performance Description: Raise your torso as high as possible. Pause briefly in this mid-range position (your torso extended) and then lower your torso under control to the start/finish position (your torso flexed) to obtain a sufficient stretch.

Training Tips:

- Avoid throwing your torso backward or snapping your head backward as you perform this exercise – movement should only occur around your hip joint and mid-section.

- If you can do 15 repetitions or more with strict form using your bodyweight, you can increase the workload on your muscles by performing the exercise with a slower speed of movement.

- This exercise may be contraindicated if you have low-back pain.

16

DESIGNING YOUR STRENGTH-TRAINING PROGRAM

You can effectively structure the framework of your strength-training program by incorporating the guidelines for improving your muscular strength that are discussed in Chapter 5 in conjunction with the exercises that are detailed in Chapters 6 - 15. But first, it's important to introduce a few additional concepts that are an integral part of designing your strength-training program.

PROGRAM DESIGN

Recall that most people can improve their muscular strength by performing a comprehensive, total-body workout that consists of no more than about 14 exercises. You should do one exercise for your hips, hamstrings, quadriceps, calves/ dorsi flexors, biceps, triceps, abdominals and lower back. Since your shoulder joint permits freedom of movement in numerous directions, you should perform two exercises for your chest, upper back (your "lats") and shoulders. If you're a "weekend warrior," a thorough workout may require a little more than 14 exercises. As an example, those who participate in a sport or activity that requires grip strength – such as softball or golf – should include one exercise in their workout to target their forearms.

There's nothing inherently wrong with doing additional exercises in order to emphasize a particular muscle. But if your level of strength begins to plateau in one or more exercises, it's probably because you're overtraining – that is, you're unable to recover from the volume of your training. Also keep in mind that placing too

much emphasis on one muscle may eventually produce abnormal development or create a muscular imbalance that can predispose you to injury. For instance, too much emphasis on your chest may lead to a round-shouldered appearance; too much emphasis on your quadriceps may make you susceptible to problems with your hamstrings.

Antagonistic Muscles

How do you know if you're doing too much work for one muscle and not enough for another? All of your muscles are arranged in such a manner that they have opposing positions and functions. As an example, your biceps on the front of your upper arm flex (or bend) your elbow and

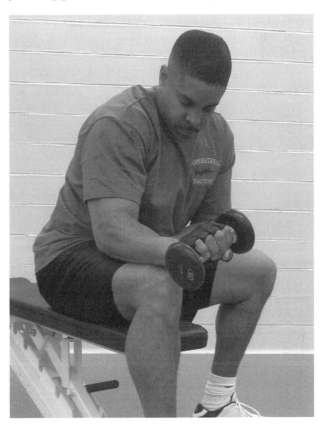

Photo 16-1: Those who participate in a sport or activity that requires grip strength – such as softball or golf – should include one exercise in their workout to target their forearms.

137

your triceps on the back of your upper arm extend (or straighten) your elbow. When one muscle acts in opposition to another, it's referred to as an "antagonist." In addition to the biceps-triceps pairing, other antagonistic muscles include your hip abductors and hip adductors; hamstrings and quadriceps; calves and dorsi flexors; chest and upper back; anterior deltoid and posterior deltoid; wrist flexors and wrist extensors; and rectus abdominis and lower back.

It's important to provide antagonistic partnerships with an equal – or nearly equal – amount of stimulus. By doing this, you'll ensure that you aren't overemphasizing a certain muscle. This, in turn, will reduce your risk of producing abnormal development and/or creating an imbalance between two muscles. Therefore, you should perform approximately the same volume of training – that is, roughly the same number of exercises, sets and repetitions – for pairs of antagonistic muscles (such as your biceps and triceps). In short, don't emphasize a particular muscle without also addressing its antagonistic counterpart with a similar volume of training.

Sequence

In designing your strength-raining program, it's worth reiterating a concept that was presented in Chapter 5. Recall that you should train your muscles from largest to smallest. Specifically, the order of exercise in a total-body workout would be as follows: hips, upper legs (hamstrings and quadriceps), lower legs (calves or dorsi flexors), torso (chest, upper back and shoulders), upper arms (biceps and triceps),

abdominals and lower back. If you do exercises for your lower arms (your forearms), you'd perform them after those for your upper arms.

The same order of exercise would still apply in a "split routine" (in which your muscles are "split" into several workouts instead of one total-body workout). In a workout that's designed to target only your chest, shoulders and triceps, for example, you should still address those muscles from largest to smallest.

Exercise Options

A summary of the exercises that are described in Chapters 6 - 15 appears in Figure 16.1. These chapters feature exercises that can be done with a variety of equipment including free weights (barbells and dumbbells) and resistance machines as well as a resistance band/cord and stability ball. Naturally, your options will differ based upon the equipment that you have available in your home.

Given the wide assortment of exercise options, the design of a strength-training routine can have almost an infinite number of possibilities. The only limits are your available equipment and your imagination.

APPLICATIONS

Based upon the information that's contained here and in Chapters 5 - 16, three sample total-body workouts are shown in Figure 16.2; similarly, a sample two-day split routine is shown in Figure 16.3. These sample workouts will give you some ideas for designing your strength-training program.

EXERCISE	MUSCLE(S) INFLUENCED	MODE
deadlift	gluteus maximus, hamstrings, quadriceps and erector spinae	BB DB TB
squat	gluteus maximus, hamstrings and quadriceps	SB
leg press	gluteus maximus, hamstrings and quadriceps	RB
lunge	gluteus maximus, hamstrings and quadriceps	BW DB SB
hip abduction	gluteus medius	AW CC
hip adduction	hip adductors	CC
prone leg curl	hamstrings	RM
seated leg curl	hamstrings	RM
leg curl	hamstrings and erector spinae	SB
leg extension	quadriceps	RM
seated calf raise	gastrocnemius and soleus	DB
standing calf raise	gastrocnemius	BW DB
dorsi flexion	dorsi flexors	CC
bench press	chest, anterior deltoids and triceps	BB DB
incline press	chest (upper), anterior deltoids and triceps	BB DB
decline press	chest (lower), anterior deltoids and triceps	BB DB
dip	chest (lower), anterior deltoids and triceps	BW
push-up	chest, anterior deltoids and triceps	BW
push-up	chest (upper), anterior deltoids and triceps	SB
bent-arm fly	chest and anterior deltoids	DB
underhand lat pulldown	upper back, biceps and forearms	CC
overhand lat pulldown	upper back, biceps and forearms	CC
chin	upper back, biceps and forearms	BW
pull-up	upper back, biceps and forearms	BW
seated row	upper back, biceps and forearms	CC
bent-over row	upper back, biceps and forearms	DB
pullover	upper back	BB DB
seated press	anterior deltoids and triceps	BB DB
lateral raise	middle deltoids and trapezius (upper)	CC DB
front raise	anterior deltoids	CC DB
bent-over raise	posterior deltoids and trapezius (middle)	CC DB
internal rotation	internal rotators	CC DB RB
external rotation	external rotators	CC DB RB
upright row	trapezius (upper), biceps and forearms	BB CC DB
shoulder shrug	trapezius (upper)	BB DB TB
scapula retraction	trapezius (middle)	CC
bicep curl	biceps and forearms	BB CC DB EZ
preacher curl	biceps and forearms	CC DB
concentration curl	biceps and forearms	CC DB
tricep extension	triceps	BB CC DB EZ
French curl	triceps	DB EZ
tricep kickback	triceps	DB
wrist flexion	wrist flexors	BB CC DB
wrist extension	wrist extensors	CC DB
wrist roller	wrist flexors, wrist extensors and anterior deltoids	RO
finger flexion	finger flexors	BB CC DB
crunch	rectus abdominis and iliopsoas	BW CC SB
knee-up	iliopsoas and rectus abdominis (lower)	BW
side bend	obliques and erector spinae	CC DB
rotary crunch	obliques and erector spinae	BW
stiff-leg deadlift	erector spinae, gluteus maximus and hamstrings	BB DB TB
back extension	erector spinae and gluteus maximus	BW SB

FIGURE 16.1: SUMMARY OF EXERCISES
MODE CODE: AW = ankle/wrist weight; BB = barbell; BW = bodyweight; CC = cable column; DB = dumbbell; EZ = EZ-curl bar; RB = resistance band/cord; RM = resistance machine; RO = roller bar; SB = stability ball; TB = trap bar

WORKOUT A	WORKOUT B	WORKOUT C
Squat (SB)	Hip Adduction (CC)	Hip Abduction (AW)
Prone Leg Curl (RM)	Seated Leg Curl (RM)	Leg Curl (SB)
Leg Extension (RM)	Leg Extension (RM)	Leg Extension (RM)
Standing Calf Raise (DB)	Dorsi Flexion (CC)	Seated Calf Raise (DB)
Dip (BW)	Bent-Arm Fly (DB)	Incline Press (BB)
Bent-Arm Fly (DB)	Bench Press (DB)	Bent-Arm Fly (DB)
Chin (BW)	Pullover (DB)	Bent-Over Row (DB)
Pullover (DB)	Seated Row (CC)	Pullover (DB)
Seated Press (BB)	Internal Rotation (RB)	Shoulder Shrug (BB)
Lateral Raise (CC)	External Rotation (RB)	Upright Row (CC)
Bicep Curl (EZ)	Preacher Curl (DB)	French Curl (EZ)
Tricep Extension (CC)	Tricep Kickback (DB)	Concentration Curl (DB)
Wrist Flexion (BB)	Wrist Extension (CC)	Wrist Roller (RO)
Side Bend (DB)	Crunch (SB)	Rotary Crunch (BW)
Back Extension (SB)	Stiff-Leg Deadlift (BB)	Back Extension (BW)

FIGURE 16.2: SAMPLE TOTAL-BODY WORKOUTS
MODE CODE: AW = ankle/wrist weight; BB = barbell; BW = bodyweight; CC = cable column; DB = dumbbell; EZ = EZ-curl bar; RB = resistance band/cord; RM = resistance machine; RO = roller bar; SB = stability ball

WORKOUT A	WORKOUT B
Deadlift (TB)	Decline Press (BB)
Seated Leg Curl (RM)	Bent-Arm Fly (DB)
Leg Extension (RM)	Seated Press (DB)
Seated Calf Raise (DB)	Shoulder Shrug (DB)
Pull-Up (BW)	Tricep Extension (EZ)
Pullover (DB)	Side Bend (CC)
Bicep Curl (BB)	Back Extension (SB)
Finger Flexion (DB)	

FIGURE 16.3: SAMPLE TWO-DAY SPLIT ROUTINE
MODE CODE: BB = barbell; BW = bodyweight; CC = cable column; DB = dumbbell; EZ = EZ-curl bar; RM = resistance machine; SB = stability ball; TB = trap bar

17

VARYING YOUR STRENGTH-TRAINING PROGRAM

At some time in your strength training, you'll undoubtedly encounter a point where your performance reaches a plateau. Quite often, this is a result of overtraining. In this case, your volume of training is so great that your muscular system is overstressed (or overworked). In effect, the demands of your training have exceeded your ability to recover. Here, you simply need to reduce your volume of training (in terms of the number of workouts, exercises and/or sets).

It's important for "weekend warriors" to understand that improvements in strength will likely be minimal during the competitive season. Although this isn't necessarily reason for alarm, the frequency of workouts and the total number of exercises may need to be reduced in order to allow for adequate recovery. In any event, the added activity of practices and competition will make it difficult to increase strength.

Sometimes, however, your performance will plateau because you're doing the same thing over and over again for lengthy periods of time. In this case, your program has become a form of unproductive manual labor that's monotonous, dull and unchallenging – a legitimate concern for many who do at-home training.

You can lessen the likelihood that this situation will occur by varying your strength-training program. Simply checking your workout card will reveal if you've reached a plateau. You should review your workout card carefully, however. If you think that you've plateaued in a certain exercise, you must consider your performance in earlier exercises of that workout. For

instance, if the resistance that you used plateaus in the bicep curl, it could be because your biceps are being exposed to increasingly heavier loads earlier in your workout when you do other exercises such as the seated row or upright row. Therefore, you must examine your entire workout in order to determine whether or not you've indeed reached a plateau.

Remember that you will not be able to improve your performance in every exercise from one workout to the next. Be that as it may, you should observe gradual increases in strength in all exercises over the course of about four or five workouts. If you're unable to make a progression in an exercise by this time – in the resistance and/or repetitions – you should vary some aspect of your strength-training program. There are several ways that this may be accomplished.

PROGRAM VARIATION

In general, you can vary three main components of your strength-training program: your workouts, exercises and sets/repetitions.

Varying Workouts

There are a number of ways that you can vary your workouts. For instance, you can change

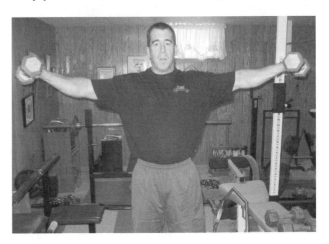

Photo 17-1: One of the easiest ways that you can integrate variety into your training is to rearrange the order in which you do your exercises for a particular muscle.

your workouts on a daily basis by doing different workouts on different days such as Workout A on Monday, Workout B on Wednesday and Workout C on Friday. You can also vary your workouts on a weekly or monthly basis. Or you can simply change them as needed. Regardless, the idea is to vary your workouts on a fairly regular basis.

Varying Exercises

You have three basic options available to vary your exercises. Specifically, you can rearrange the order, change the equipment and alternate the exercises.

Rearrange the Order

One of the easiest ways that you can integrate variety into your training is to rearrange the order in which you do your exercises for a particular muscle. Suppose, for example, that you desire a change in the way that you train your shoulders. If you've been doing the seated press followed by the lateral raise, you can incorporate variety by simply switching the two exercises. In other words, you can perform the lateral raise first and the seated press second.

Keep in mind that whenever you change the order in which you do your exercises, you must adjust the levels of resistance. So if you do the lateral raise first (instead of second), your shoulders will be fresh and, therefore, you should increase the resistance in that exercise. And if you do the seated press second (instead of first), your shoul-

ders will be fatigued and, therefore, you must decrease the resistance in that exercise.

An additional possibility is to rearrange the order in which you train your muscles. Rather than go from chest to upper back ("lats") to shoulders, you might start with your shoulders, proceed to your upper back and then finish with your chest. So a six-exercise sequence for your torso of bench press, bent-arm fly, seated row, pullover, seated press and lateral raise could be changed to lateral raise, seated press, pullover, seated row, bent-arm fly and bench press. Once again, remember that you'll need to adjust the levels of resistance any time that you rearrange the order of exercises.

Change the Equipment

Another way that you can vary the exercises is to change the equipment that you use. Say that you've been doing the bicep curl with a barbell for quite some time and, consequently, desire a change of pace. In this situation, you can perform the bicep curl with another type of equipment such as an EZ-curl bar, dumbbells or a cable column. Obviously, the extent to which you can change the equipment depends upon what you have available for at-home training.

Alternate the Exercises

A third means of varying exercises is to alternate them with other ones that employ the same muscles. Consider this: The seated row involves your upper back, biceps and forearms. And so do other rowing, chinning and pulling movements such as the underhand lat pulldown, overhand lat pulldown, chin, pull-up and bent-over row. Therefore, any of these exercises are potential substitutes for the seated row. Once again, the availability of equipment will determine how much you can alternate your exercises.

Besides providing for variety, periodically alternating your exercises (and/or equipment) has another advantage: It allows you to train your muscles through different ranges of motion. In this way, you can target your muscles in a more complete and comprehensive manner.

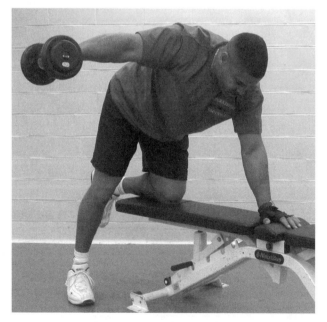

Photo 17-2: Besides providing for variety, periodically alternating your exercises (and/or equipment) allows you to train your muscles through different ranges of motion.

Varying Sets/Repetitions

A final component of your strength-training program that you can vary is the way that you do a set which essentially is the way that you do a repetition. Ordinarily, repetitions are performed in a bilateral manner – that is, with both limbs at the same time. You can, however, do at least five other variations including negative-only, negative-accentuated, unilateral, modified-cadence and extended-pause repetitions.

But a few words of caution: Although the upcoming ways of varying a repetition may sound simple, a reasonably high level of skill is required to do them in a manner that's safe and effective. Because of this, you shouldn't attempt to implement any of these advanced applications in your program until you can demonstrate proper technique when you perform repetitions in a bilateral fashion.

Negative-Only Repetitions

You can perform your repetitions in a negative-only manner by having another person (a "spotter") raise the resistance and you lower it. Essentially, the spotter does the positive (or concentric) work and the lifter does the negative (or eccentric) work. In the bench press, for example, you'd perform a set of negative-only repetitions as follows: The spotter lifts the bar out of the uprights and you hold it in the start/finish position (your arms almost fully extended). After the spotter releases the bar, you lower the weight under control until it touches the middle part of your chest. Then, the spotter would raise the bar off your chest to the start/finish position. This procedure would be repeated for the desired number of repetitions.

Keep in mind that your eccentric (or negative) strength is always greater than your concentric (or positive) strength in the same exercise. In other words, you can always lower a greater amount of resistance than you can raise (again, in the same exercise). This means that you can use more resistance for repetitions that are done in a negative-only manner than you can for repetitions that are done in a traditional manner. How much more? If you're performing negative-only repetitions for the first time, start with about 10% more resistance than you're normally capable of handling. So if you most recently used 150 pounds on an exercise in the traditional manner, increase the resistance by about 15 pounds – that is, to 165 pounds – for a set of negative-only repetitions. If you attain the maximum number of negative-only repetitions, you should increase the resistance for your next workout.

To achieve the best results, negative-only repetitions should be done slowly. In general, each negative-only repetition should be performed in about 6 - 8 seconds. Ranges of time that will work well for most individuals are about 90 - 120 seconds for a hip exercise, 60 - 90 seconds for a leg exercise and 40 - 70 seconds for a torso exercise. Based upon these windows of time, then, an eight-second negative-only repetition would translate into repetition ranges of about 11 - 15 for the hips, 8 - 11 for the legs and 5 - 9 for the torso.

Performing negative-only repetitions is extremely demanding. For this reason, they shouldn't be done in any given exercise more than once per week.

Negative-Accentuated Repetitions

The major disadvantage of doing negative-only repetitions is that at least one other person is almost always required to lift the weight. For the most part, you can only perform negative-only repetitions without needing assistance from someone else in a handful of exercises that involve your bodyweight as resistance such as push-ups, dips, chins, pull-ups and crunches. In the chin, for example, you'd perform negative-only repetitions as follows: Step or climb up to the mid-range position (your arms flexed) and pause briefly. Lower your body under control to the start/finish position (your arms fully extended). This procedure would be repeated for the desired number of repetitions.

But again, other than several exercises that involve your bodyweight, you need help in order to do negative-only repetitions. The value of negative-accentuated repetitions is that they emphasize the eccentric component of an exercise yet they can be performed without any assistance from another individual. When doing negative-accentuated repetitions, both limbs share the positive work but only one limb does the negative work. In other words, the resistance is raised with two arms or legs and then lowered with only one arm or leg.

Although it's impossible to perform negative-accentuated repetitions with a barbell, you can use this technique to do several exercises with a dumbbell. In the bicep curl, for example, you'd perform a set of negative-accentuated repetitions as follows: Hold the dumbbell in your right hand and straighten your right arm. Grasp your right wrist with your left hand. Using both arms, raise the dumbbell to the mid-range position (your arms flexed) and pause briefly. Move your left hand away from your right wrist and hold the dumbbell momentarily with your right arm. Lower the dumbbell under control to the start/finish position (your arm fully extended) with your right arm. Raise the resistance to the mid-range position with both arms and continue the preceding sequence using your right arm to lower the dumbbell. This procedure would be repeated for the desired number of repetitions. (Note: In this case, you'd lower the dumbbell with the same arm for the entire set and then repeat the exercise for the other side of your body.)

You can also do negative-accentuated repetitions with many resistance machines. In the leg extension, for example, you'd perform a set of negative-accentuated repetitions as follows: Using both legs, raise the resistance to the mid-range position (your legs fully extended) and pause briefly. Move your left leg away from the roller pad and hold the resistance momentarily with your right leg. Lower the resistance under control to the start/finish position (your leg flexed) with your right leg. Raise the resistance to the mid-range position with both legs and continue the preceding sequence using your left leg to lower the resistance. This procedure would be repeated for the desired number of repetitions. (Note: In this case, you'd lower the weight by alternating your right and left legs.)

Similar to negative-only repetitions, the resistance should be lowered in about 6 - 8 seconds. As a starting point, use about 70% of the resistance that you normally handle in the traditional fashion. So if you last used 100 pounds on an exercise, begin with 70 pounds for negative-accentuated repetitions. In the case of negative-accentuated exercise, appropriate repetition ranges for most individuals are about 15 - 20 for the hips, 10 - 15 for the legs and 6 - 12 for the torso. (Note that these are the total repetitions for both limbs, not the total repetitions for each limb.)

One final point: It's important that you maintain a stable position when doing negative-accentuated repetitions. In particular, you should avoid twisting or turning your torso.

Unilateral Repetitions

As a variation in the repetition style, many exercises can be done unilaterally (one limb at a time). Besides adding variety to your training, unilateral repetitions are advisable for those who have an injury on one side of the body or a strength imbalance between one side of the body and the other. They're also recommended for individuals with hypertension (high blood pressure).

Modified-Cadence Repetitions

Another option is to vary the cadence or speed with which you normally perform your repetitions. One cadence that has received a great deal of national attention is the SuperSlow® Protocol which was introduced by Ken Hutchins in the early 1980s. The basic cadence for SuperSlow® repetitions is to raise the resistance in 10 seconds and lower it in 5 seconds (or 10/5). Other popular variations of repetition speed include 4/4, 8/8 and 10/10. A single set consisting of one 30/30 repetition can also be done – in other words, one repetition that takes 60 seconds to complete. Keep in mind that you'll need to adjust your repetition ranges any time that you modify the duration of a repetition.

Extended-Pause Repetitions

It's important to pause briefly – about one second or so – in the mid-range position of each repetition. There are at least three reasons for emphasizing the mid-range position. First, it enables you to strengthen an otherwise weak position in your range of motion. Second, it allows you to focus on your muscles when they're fully contracted. Third, it permits a smooth transition between raising and lowering the weight.

As a repetition variation, the brief pause in the mid-range position can be done for a slightly longer duration – perhaps in three or four seconds. Using this technique is also an excellent tool to incorporate in the initial stages of training in order to understand the concept – and

Photo 17-3: As a variation in the repetition style, many exercises can be done unilaterally (one limb at a time).

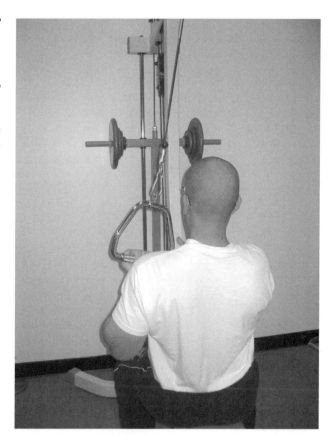

value – of pausing in the mid-range position. Once again, remember that you'll need to adjust your repetition ranges any time that you modify the duration of a repetition.

Note that an extended pause in the mid-range position essentially involves a mild isometric contraction that tends to elevate blood pressure beyond that which is normally encountered. As such, individuals who have hypertension shouldn't use this technique.

APPLICATIONS

You can inject excitement into your at-home training by incorporating variety. Individuals can vary an entire workout or simply one or two aspects of it such as the exercises or sets/repetitions. For instance, refer to the sample workouts that are given in Chapter 16 (Figures 16.2 and 16.3). As you can see, simply varying exercises can produce significant changes in the complexion of workouts.

How often should you vary your strength-training program? For the most part, this depends upon the individual. But in general, those who are just initiating a strength-training program or haven't been doing one for too long prob-

ably will not require much variety; those who are more experienced will need to vary their programs on a regular basis.

As they say, "Variety is the spice of life." Clearly, the same holds true for strength training.

18

FUELING YOUR ACTIVE LIFESTYLE

Nutrition is the process by which you select, consume, digest, absorb and utilize food. Unfortunately, this facet of an active lifestyle is either inadequately addressed or entirely overlooked.

Implementing good nutritional practices has several purposes. First of all, proper nutrition plays a critical role in your capacity to perform at optimal levels and to expedite recovery. Clearly, your ability to fully recuperate after an exhaustive activity directly affects your future performances and the intensity of your training. Your nutritional habits are also a factor in the development of your physical attributes such as your muscular strength and aerobic fitness.

As a result, having knowledge of proper nutrition is very critical. You can improve your nutritional skills by recognizing the desirable food sources, understanding the recommended intakes of those food sources and realizing the caloric contributions of the various nutrients. In addition, becoming familiar with your caloric needs can provide support for nutritional planning. Moreover, knowing what foods/fluids to consume before and after vigorous activity will help to maximize your training. Finally, having knowledge of proper nutrition will assist you in determining whether or not supplements are warranted.

THE NUTRIENTS

Everything that you do requires energy. The energy is obtained through the foods (or nutrients) that you consume and is measured in calories. Essentially, the foods that you eat serve as a fuel for your body. Food is also necessary for the growth, maintenance and repair of biological tissues such as muscle and bone.

Foods are composed of six nutrients: carbohydrates, protein, fat, water, vitamins and minerals. These main constituents of food can be grouped as either macronutrients or micronutrients. In order to be considered nutritious, your food intake must contain the recommended amounts of the macronutrients as well as appropriate levels of the micronutrients. No single food satisfies this requirement. As a result, variety is the key to a balanced diet. (Here and in other discussions that follow, the term "diet" simply refers to a normal food intake, not a specialized regimen of eating.)

The Macronutrients

As the name implies, macronutrients are needed in relatively large amounts. Three macronutrients – carbohydrates, protein and fat – provide you with calories and, therefore, a supply of energy. Although it has no calories, water is also categorized as a macronutrient because it's needed in considerable quantities.

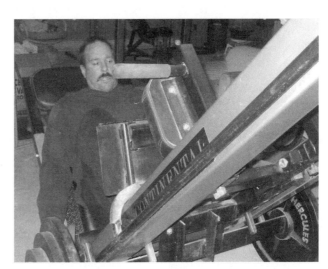

Photo 18-1: The primary fuction of carbohydrates (or "carbs") is to furnish you with energy, especially during intense activity.

147

Carbohydrates

The primary function of carbohydrates (or "carbs") is to furnish you with energy, especially during intense activity. The body breaks down carbohydrates into blood glucose (or "blood sugar"). Glucose can be used as an immediate form of energy during an activity or stored as glycogen in your liver and muscles for future use. Highly conditioned muscles can stockpile more glycogen than poorly conditioned muscles. If your glycogen stores are depleted, you'll feel overwhelmingly exhausted. For this reason, having greater glycogen stores can give you a significant physiological advantage. It makes a great deal of sense, therefore, that your diet should be carbohydrate-based. In fact, at least 65% of your daily calories should be in the form of carbohydrates.

Carbohydrates are classified as either "simple" (which are sugars such as table sugar and honey) or "complex" (which are starches such as bread). Foods that are high in carbohydrates include potatoes, cereals, pancakes, waffles, breads, bagels, spaghetti, macaroni, rice, grains, fruits and vegetables.

Protein

Protein is necessary for the growth, maintenance and repair of biological tissues, particularly muscle tissue. In addition, protein regulates water balance and transports other nutrients. Protein can also be used as an energy source in the event that adequate carbohydrates and fat aren't available.

When proteins are ingested as foods, they're broken down into their basic building blocks: amino acids. The body can manufacture most of the 22 known amino acids. Eight (or nine in the case of children and certain adults) must be provided in the diet and are termed "essential amino acids." When a food contains all of the essential amino acids in amounts that facilitate the growth and repair of muscle tissue, it's deemed a "complete protein." In addition, such foods are considered to have a high "biological value" meaning that a large portion of the protein is absorbed and retained. The biological value is an index in which all protein sources are compared to egg whites because they're the most complete protein. (Egg whites have a biological value of 100).

All animal proteins – with the exception of gelatin – are complete proteins and, as a result, have a high biological value. Conversely, the protein found in vegetables and other sources is considered to be an "incomplete protein" – having a low biological value – because it doesn't include all of the essential amino acids. A white potato, for instance, has a biological value of 34.

Approximately 15% of your daily calories should be from protein. Good sources of this macronutrient are beef, pork, fish, poultry, eggs, liver, dry beans and dairy products.

Fat

It may be difficult to believe but fat is actually vital to a balanced diet. First, fat serves as a major source of energy during low-intensity activities such as sleeping, reading and walking. Second, fat helps in the transportation and absorption of certain vitamins. Third, fat adds substantial flavor to foods. This makes food much more appetizing – and also explains why fat is craved so much.

Foods that are high in fat include butter, cheese, margarine, meat, nuts, dairy products and cooking oils. Animal fats – such as butter, lard and the fat in meats – are referred to as "saturated fats" and contribute to heart disease; vegetable fats – such as corn, olive and peanut oils – are dubbed "unsaturated fats" and are less harmful. (At room temperature, saturated fats tend to be solid while unsaturated fats are usually liquid.)

There's really no need for you to add extra fatty food to your diet in order to obtain adequate fat. If anything, most people consume far too much fat. The fact is that fat often accompanies carbohydrate and protein choices. In addition, foods are often prepared in such a way that the fat content is elevated. For example, baked potatoes have a negligible amount of fat – barely a trace of their calories; french-fried potatoes, on the other hand, have a considerable amount of fat – approximately one half of their calories.

At most, about 20% of your daily calories should be composed of fat. Keep in mind that this allotment of fat – as well as that of carbohydrates and protein – is to be distributed over the course of the day. So, there's nothing wrong with eating a food that's more than 20% fat as long as you offset this particular choice by consuming other foods throughout the day that have a lower fat content.

Water

Since it's needed in rather large quantities, water is usually classified as a macronutrient. Water doesn't have any calories or provide you with any energy but it does play major roles in your body. For one thing, water lubricates your joints and regulates your body temperature. Also, water helps carry nutrients to the cells and waste products from the cells. Incredibly, almost two thirds of your bodyweight is water.

The best sources of water are milk, fruits, fruit juices, vegetables, soup and, of course, water. You should consume about 16 ounces of water for every pound of bodyweight that you lose during your training.

The Micronutrients

Vitamins and minerals are classified as micronutrients because they're required in somewhat small amounts. Neither of these nutrients supplies you with any calories or energy. But vitamins and minerals have many other important functions. (It's well beyond the scope of this chapter to provide you with an extensive overview of the functions and sources of vitamins and minerals. For more detailed information, you're encouraged to pursue other sources.)

Vitamins

The Polish chemist Casimir Funk coined the term "vitamine" in 1912. Vitamins are potent compounds that are required in very minute quantities. They occur in a wide variety of foods, especially in fruits and vegetables. You can obtain an adequate intake of vitamins from a balanced diet that contains a variety of foods. Even though vitamins aren't a source of energy, they perform many different functions that are vital to an active lifestyle.

Vitamins can be grouped as either fat-soluble or water-soluble.

Fat-Soluble Vitamins

The four fat-soluble vitamins – vitamins A, D, E and K – require proper amounts of fat to be present before transportation and absorption can take place. Excessive amounts of fat-soluble vitamins are stored in the body.

Here's a brief listing of their functions and sources:

- Vitamin A (retinol) is required for normal vision (especially at night) and promotes bone growth, healthy hair, skin and teeth. Organ meats, dairy products, fish, eggs, carrots, spinach and sweet potatoes are good sources of this vitamin.

- Vitamin D (calciferol) enhances calcium absorption and is vital for strong bones and teeth. The "sunshine vitamin" can be found in fish, fortified milk products and cereals, dairy products and egg yolks.

- Vitamin E (tocopherol) acts as an antioxidant, aids in the formation of red blood cells and helps to maintain the muscles and other biological tissues. Once known as "the vitamin in search of a disease," good sources of it are poultry, seafood, eggs, vegetable oils, nuts, fruits, vegetables and meats.

- Vitamin K assists in blood clotting and bone metabolism. It's found in green leafy vegetables, brussel sprouts, cabbage, potatoes, plant oils, oats, margarine and organ meats.

Water-Soluble Vitamins

The eight B vitamins – biotin, cobalamin, folate, niacin, pantothenic acid, pyridoxine, riboflavin and thiamine – and vitamin C are considered to be water-soluble vitamins because they're found in foods that have a naturally high content of water. There's minimal storage of water-soluble vitamins in the body – excess amounts are generally excreted in the urine.

Their functions and sources are summarized as follows:

- Biotin helps to synthesize glycogen, amino acids and fat. Rich sources of biotin are liver, fruits, vegetables, nuts, eggs, poultry and meats.

- Cobalamin (B_{12}) forms and regulates red blood cells, prevents anemia and maintains a healthy nervous system. This vitamin can be found in fortified cereals, meats, fish, poultry and dairy products.

- Folate (folic acid and folacin) is needed to manufacture red blood cells and aids in the metabolism of amino acids. Enriched cereal grains, fruits, dark green leafy vegetables, meats, fish, liver, poultry, enriched and whole-grain breads and fortified cereals are good sources of folate.

- Niacin (B_3) promotes normal appetite, digestion and proper nerve function and is required for energy metabolism. It's found in meats, fish, poultry, eggs, potatoes, enriched and whole-grain breads and bread products, orange juice, peanuts and fortified cereals.

- Pantothenic acid (B_5) helps in the metabolism of carbohydrates, protein and fat. Good sources of this vitamin are chicken, beef, potatoes, oats, cereals, tomato products, liver, kidney, yeast, egg yolks, broccoli and whole grains.

- Pyridoxine (B_6) assists in the formation of red blood cells and the metabolism of carbohydrates, protein and fat. Fortified cereals, organ meats, lean meats, poultry, fish, eggs, milk, vegetables, nuts and bananas are rich sources of this vitamin.

- Riboflavin (B_2) aids in the maintenance of skin, mucous membranes and nervous structures. This vitamin is found in organ meats, poultry, beef, lamb, fish, milk, dark green leafy vegetables, bread products and fortified cereals.

- Thiamine (B_1) maintains a healthy nervous system and heart and helps to metabolize carbohydrates and amino acids. Good sources of thiamine are enriched, fortified and whole-grain products, bread and bread products, ready-to-eat cereals, meats, poultry, fish, liver and eggs.

- Vitamin C (ascorbic acid) promotes healing, helps in the absorption of iron and the maintenance and repair of connective tissues, bones, teeth and cartilage. Citrus fruits, tomatoes, tomato juice, potatoes, brussel sprouts, cauliflower, broccoli, strawberries, watermelon, cabbage and spinach are rich sources of vitamin C.

Minerals

Minerals are found in tiny amounts in foods. Like vitamins, nearly all of the minerals that you need can be obtained with an ordinary intake of foods.

Minerals can be divided into two subcategories: macrominerals and microminerals.

Macrominerals

As the name implies, macrominerals are required in relatively large amounts – specifically, more than 250 milligrams per day. The macrominerals are calcium, chloride, magnesium, phosphorus, potassium, sodium and sulfur.

Here's a brief overview of their functions and sources:

- Calcium is essential in blood clotting, muscle contraction, nerve transmission and the formation of bones and teeth. Rich sources of this mineral are milk, cheese, yogurt, oysters, broccoli and spinach.

- Chloride is an electrolyte that regulates body fluids in to and out of the cells and helps to maintain a proper acid-base (pH) balance. It's found in table salt, milk, canned vegetables and animal foods.

- Magnesium is essential for healthy nerve and muscle function and bone formation. Green leafy vegetables, nuts, meats, poultry, fish, oysters, starches, milk and beans are good sources of magnesium.

- Phosphorus maintains pH, helps in energy production and is essential for every metabolic process in the body. Good sources are milk, yogurt, ice cream, cheese, peas, meats, poultry, fish and eggs.

- Potassium is an electrolyte that regulates body fluids in to and out of the cells and promotes proper muscular contraction and the transmission of nerve impulses. This mineral is found in citrus fruits, bananas, deep yellow vegetables and potatoes.

- Sodium is an electrolyte that regulates body fluids in to and out of the cells, transmits nerve impulses, maintains normal blood pressure and is involved in muscular contraction. Table salt, milk, canned vegetables and animal foods are good sources of sodium.

- Sulfur is needed to make hair and nails. It's found in beef, peanuts, clams and wheat germ.

Microminerals

As might be suspected, microminerals are needed in relatively small amounts – specifically, less than 20 milligrams per day. The microminerals are chromium, copper, fluoride,

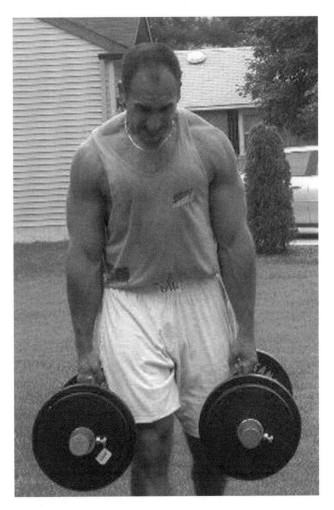

Photo 18-2: Your caloric needs are determined by several factors such as your age, gender, size, body composition, metabolic rate and level of activity.

iodine, iron, manganese, molybdenum, selenium and zinc. (A number of other minerals – including arsenic, boron, cobalt, lithium, nickel, silicon, tin and vanadium – are probably essential in very small amounts but their roles in the human body are unclear and recommended intakes haven't been established.)

This is a quick rundown of the functions and sources of the microminerals:

- Chromium functions in the metabolism of carbohydrates and fat and helps to maintain levels of blood glucose. Meats, poultry, fish and peanuts are good sources of chromium.
- Copper stimulates the absorption of iron and has a role in the formation of red blood cells, connective tissues and nerve fibers. Good sources are organ meats, seafood, nuts, beans, whole-grain products and cocoa products.
- Fluoride prevents dental caries and stimulates the formation of new bones. This mineral is found in fluoridated water, teas and marine fish.
- Iodine is necessary for proper functioning of the thyroid gland and prevents goiter and cretinism. Seafood, processed foods and iodized salt are good sources of this mineral.
- Iron is involved in the manufacture of hemoglobin and myoglobin (two proteins that transport oxygen to the tissues) and has a role in normal immune function. It's found in liver, fruits, vegetables, fortified bread and grain products, meats, poultry and shellfish.
- Manganese is involved in the formation of bones and the metabolism of carbohydrates. Good sources of manganese are nuts, legumes, coffee, tea and whole grains.
- Molybdenum helps to regulate the storage of iron. Dark green leafy vegetables, legumes, grain products, nuts and organ meats are good sources of this mineral.
- Selenium protects cell membranes. It's found in organ meats, chicken, seafood, whole-grain

cereals and milk.

- Zinc has a role in the repair and growth of biological tissues. Good sources of this mineral are fortified cereals, meats, poultry, eggs and seafood.

DAILY SERVINGS

Consuming an assortment of foods helps to ensure that you've obtained adequate amounts of carbohydrates, protein and fat along with sufficient quantities of vitamins and minerals. According to the U. S. Department of Agriculture (USDA) Food Guide that was made public in January 2005, a variety of daily foods should include an appropriate number of servings from these six food groups:

- Fruit
- Vegetable
- Grain
- Meat and Beans
- Milk
- Oils

The exact number of servings that are suitable for you is contingent upon your caloric (energy) needs. Your caloric needs depend upon a number of factors, including your age, gender, size, body composition, metabolic rate and level of activity.

RECOMMENDED DIETARY ALLOWANCES

First published in 1943 and updated regularly, the Recommended Dietary Allowances (RDAs) were developed by the Food and Nutrition Board of the National Academy of Sciences/National Research Council. The RDAs are set by first determining the "floor" below which deficiency occurs and then the "ceiling" above which harm occurs. A margin of safety is included in the RDAs to meet the requirements of nearly all healthy people. In fact, the RDAs are designed to cover the biological needs of *97.5% of the population*. In other words, the RDAs exceed what most people require in order to meet the needs of those who have the highest requirements. So, the RDAs don't represent minimum standards. And failing to consume the recommended amounts doesn't necessarily indicate that a person has a dietary deficiency. (The RDAs of selected vitamins and minerals for men and women aged 19 - 70 are given in Tables 18.1 and 18.2, respectively.)

CALORIC CONTRIBUTIONS

As mentioned previously, three macronutrients – carbohydrates, protein and fat – furnish you with calories, albeit in different amounts. Carbohydrates and protein yield four calories per gram (cal/g). Fat is the most concentrated form of energy, containing nine cal/g. Armed with this information, you can determine the caloric contributions for each of the three energy-providing macronutrients in any food – provided that you know how many grams of each macronutrient are in a serving.

As an example, consider a snack food such as Fritos® Brand Original Corn Chips (Frito-Lay, Incorporated). Examining the nutrition facts label reveals that a one-ounce serving of this product contains 15 grams of carbohydrates, 2 grams of protein and 10 grams of fat. To find the exact number of calories that are supplied by each macronutrient, simply multiply its number of grams per serving by its corresponding energy

yield. In this example, each serving of the food has 60 calories from carbohydrates [15 g x 4 cal/g], 8 calories from protein [2 g x 4 cal/g] and 90 calories from fat [10 g x 9 cal/g]. Therefore, this food has a total of 158 calories per serving (which is rounded up to 160 on the nutrition facts label). As can be seen, this product has 50% more grams of carbohydrates than fat (15 compared to 10) – yet nearly 57% of the calories (90 of the 158) are furnished by fat. Moreover, consuming the entire contents of the 2.5-ounce bag will contribute 25 grams of fat – or 225 calories from fat – to your caloric budget.

Compare this to Baked Lays® Potato Crisps, another snack food by the same manufacturer. A one-ounce serving of this product has 23 grams of carbohydrates, 2 grams of protein and 1.5 grams of fat. Each serving of this food contains 92 calories from carbohydrates [23 g x 4 cal/g], 8 calories from protein [2 g x 4 cal/g] and 13.5 calories from fat [1.5 g x 9 cal/g]. So this food has a total of 113.5 calories per serving (which is rounded down to 110 on the nutrition facts label). This particular product, then, has more than 15 times as many grams of carbohydrates than fat (23 compared to 1.5) – and only 11.9% of the calories (13.5 of the 113.5) are supplied by fat. Furthermore, consuming 2.5 ounces of this product will add a mere 3.75 grams of fat – or 33.75 calories from fat – to your caloric budget.

Knowing the different caloric contributions of the macronutrients is also helpful in understanding information about fat content on the packaging of a product that could easily be misinterpreted. Case in point: A package that proclaims a product to be "99% fat free" means that it's 99% fat free by weight, not by calories. How critical is this distinction? Very. Placing one gram of fat into 99 grams of water forms a product that – in terms of weight – is "99% fat free." But since water has no calories, this particular "99% fat free" product would actually be – in terms of calories – 100% fat.

Although the preceding example was hypothetical, the fact is that this discrepancy actually occurs on the packaging of many products. Here are four illustrations of real products:

- A can of College Inn® Chicken Broth (H. J. Heinz Company) states that it's "99% fat free." But one serving of this product (241 grams)

VITAMIN (units)	MEN				
	9-13	14-18	19-30	31-50	51-70
Vitamin A (mcg)	600	900	900	900	900
Vitamin D (mcg)	5	5	5	5	10
Vitamin E (mg)	11	15	15	15	15
Vitamin K (mcg)	60	75	120	120	120
Biotin (mcg)	20	25	30	30	30
Choline (mg)	375	550	550	550	550
Folate (mcg)	300	400	400	400	400
Niacin (mg)	12	16	16	16	16
Pantothenic Acid (mg)	4	5	5	5	5
Riboflavin (mg)	0.9	1.3	1.3	1.3	1.3
Thiamin (mg)	0.9	1.2	1.2	1.2	1.2
Pyridoxine (mg)	1.0	1.3	1.3	1.3	1.7
Cobalamin (mcg)	1.8	2.4	2.4	2.4	2.4
Vitamin C (mg)	45	75	90	90	90

VITAMIN (units)	WOMEN					Pregnancy		Lactation	
	9-13	14-18	19-30	31-50	51-70	19-30	31-50	19-30	31-50
Vitamin A (mcg)	600	700	700	700	700	770	770	1,300	1,300
Vitamin D (mcg)	5	5	5	5	10	5	5	5	5
Vitamin E (mg)	11	15	15	15	15	15	15	19	19
Vitamin K (mcg)	60	75	90	90	90	90	90	90	90
Biotin (mcg)	20	25	30	30	30	30	30	35	35
Choline (mg)	375	400	425	425	425	450	450	550	550
Folate (mcg)	300	400	400	400	400	600	600	500	500
Niacin (mg)	12	14	14	14	14	18	18	17	17
Pantothenic Acid (mg)	4	5	5	5	5	6	6	7	7
Riboflavin (mg)	0.9	1.0	1.1	1.1	1.1	1.4	1.4	1.6	1.6
Thiamin (mg)	0.9	1.0	1.1	1.1	1.1	1.4	1.4	1.4	1.4
Pyridoxine (mg)	1.0	1.2	1.3	1.3	1.5	1.9	1.9	2.0	2.0
Cobalamin (mcg)	1.8	2.4	2.4	2.4	2.4	2.6	2.6	2.8	2.8
Vitamin C (mg)	45	65	75	75	75	85	85	120	120

TABLE 18.1: RECOMMENDED DIETARY ALLOWANCES (RDAs) OF SELECTED VITAMINS FOR MEN AND WOMEN AGED 19 - 70

MINERAL (units)	MEN				
	9-13	14-18	19-30	31-50	51-70
Calcium (mg)	1,300	1,300	1,000	1,000	1,200
Chromium (mcg)	25	35	35	35	30
Copper (mcg)	700	890	900	900	900
Fluoride (mg)	2	3	4	4	4
Iodine (mcg)	120	150	150	150	150
Iron (mg)	8	11	8	8	8
Magnesium (mg)	240	410	400	420	420
Manganese (mg)	1.9	2.2	2.3	2.3	2.3
Molybdenum (mcg)	34	43	45	45	45
Phosphorus (mg)	1,250	1,250	700	700	700
Selenium (mcg)	40	55	55	55	55
Zinc (mg)	8	11	11	11	11

MINERAL (units)	WOMEN					Pregnancy		Lactation	
	9-13	14-18	19-30	31-50	51-70	19-30	31-50	19-30	31-50
Calcium (mg)	1,300	1,300	1,000	1,000	1,200	1,000	1,000	1,000	1,000
Chromium (mcg)	21	24	25	25	20	30	30	45	45
Copper (mcg)	700	890	900	900	900	1,000	1,000	1,300	1,300
Fluoride (mg)	2	3	3	3	3	3	3	3	3
Iodine (mcg)	120	150	150	150	150	220	220	290	290
Iron (mg)	8	15	18	18	8	27	27	9	9
Magnesium (mg)	240	360	310	320	320	350	360	310	320
Manganese (mg)	1.6	1.6	1.8	1.8	1.8	2.0	2.0	2.6	2.6
Molybdenum (mcg)	34	43	45	45	45	50	50	50	50
Phosphorus (mg)	1,250	1,250	700	700	700	700	700	700	700
Selenium (mcg)	40	55	55	55	55	60	60	70	70
Zinc (mg)	8	9	8	8	8	11	11	12	12

TABLE 18.2: RECOMMENDED DIETARY ALLOWANCES (RDAs) OF SELECTED MINERALS FOR MEN AND WOMEN AGED 19 - 70

has 9 calories of which 9 are from fat – meaning that it's 100% fat.

- A package of Hershey®'s Chocolate Drink (Hershey® Foods Corporation) states that it's "99% fat free." But one serving of this product (eight ounces) has 129 calories of which 9 are from fat – meaning that it's 6.98% fat.

- A package of Black Bear of the Black Forest™ Gourmet Cooked Ham (Black Bear Enterprises, Incorporated) states that it's "98% fat free." But one serving of this product (two ounces) has 49 calories of which 9 are from fat – meaning that it's 18.37% fat.

- A package of Oscar Mayer® Dinner Ham (Oscar Mayer Foods) notes that it's "96% fat free." But one serving of this product (three ounces) has 83 calories of which 27 are from fat – meaning that it's 32.53% fat.

With the exception of the chicken broth, the percentages of fat calories for these four products aren't terribly bad. But it's certainly a far cry from how the percentages on the package can be interpreted.

ESTIMATING YOUR CALORIC BUDGET

As mentioned earlier, your caloric needs are determined by several factors such as your age, gender, size, body composition, metabolic rate and level of activity. For a quick and reasonably accurate estimate of your daily caloric needs, the U. S. Department of Agriculture suggests multiplying your bodyweight by a number that corresponds to your approximate level of activity. Essentially, this number represents your energy requirements in calories per pound of your bodyweight (cal/lb). For women, the values are 14 if sedentary, 18 if moderately active and 22 if very active; for men, the numbers are 16, 21 and 26. To illustrate, a 180-pound man who's moderately active requires about 3,780 calories per day (cal/day) to meet his energy needs [180 lb x 21 cal/lb].

Once you've estimated your caloric budget, you can determine how many of these calories should come from carbohydrates, protein and fat. Using the previous example, someone who requires about 3,780 cal/day should consume roughly 614.25 grams of carbohydrates [3,780 cal/day x 0.65 ÷ 4 cal/g], 141.75 grams of protein [3,780 cal/day x 0.15 ÷ 4 cal/g] and 84.0

grams of fat [3,780 cal/day x 0.20 ÷ 9 cal/g]. Note that these numbers are based upon a diet that consists of 65% carbohydrates, 15% protein and 20% fat.

PRE-ACTIVITY FOODS/FUELS

Before an activity, any foods that you consume should satisfy your hunger, ready your body with fuel for your upcoming effort and relax your psychological state. Because your body prefers to use carbohydrates for energy during intense activity, it makes sense that any foods consumed prior to an activity should be high in that macronutrient.

That being said, you should avoid eating carbohydrates that cause a sharp increase in your blood glucose. Here's why: In response to a high level of blood glucose, the body increases its level of blood insulin to maintain a stable internal environment. As a result of this biochemical balancing, blood glucose is sharply reduced. This leads to hypoglycemia (or "low blood sugar") which decreases the availability of blood glucose as a fuel and causes an individual to feel severely fatigued. Although this condition is usually temporary, it remains an important consideration. The idea, then, is to consume foods that elevate or maintain blood glucose without triggering a dramatic response by blood insulin.

At one time, it was thought that simple carbohydrates (sugars) increase blood glucose more rapidly than complex carbohydrates (starches). A more recent trend of thought has been to consider the Glycemic Index (GI) of a food. The GI dates back to 1981 when it was conceptualized by a group of scientists as a way to help determine which foods were best for people with diabetes. The GI is a system of quantifying the carbohydrates in foods based upon how they affect blood glucose. A value is assigned to a food that correlates to the magnitude of the increase in blood glucose. For instance, a food with a GI of 25 means that it elevates blood glucose to a level that's 25% as great as consuming the same amount of pure glucose (which has a GI of 100). Incidentally, the GI isn't related to portion size. So, the GI is the same whether you consume 10 grams of a particular food or 110 grams. The number of calories, of course, would differ according to the size of the portion.

Preceding an activity, it's best to consume foods that are high in carbohydrates with a low GI. These foods help to keep your blood glucose within a desirable range. Don't simply assume that a sugary food raises blood glucose more than a starchy food. Indeed, honey has a lower GI than a bagel and, given these two options, would be a better choice prior to an activity. Foods with a relatively low GI include milk, apple juice, orange juice, tomato juice, apples, cherries, grapefruit, grapes, oranges, pears, plums, yogurt, macaroni, plain pizza, spaghetti, beans, nuts and oatmeal. (It's well beyond the scope of this chapter to provide you with an extensive overview of foods and their GIs. For more detailed information, you're encouraged to pursue other sources.)

Water is perhaps the best liquid for you to drink before training or competing. Your fluid intake should be enough to guarantee optimal hydration during the activity.

The timing of the pre-activity meal is also crucial. To ensure that the digestive process doesn't impair your performance, you should eat your pre-activity meal at least three hours prior to training or competing. In short, the pre-activity meal should include foods that are familiar to you and are well tolerated – preferably carbohydrates with a low GI.

POST-ACTIVITY FOODS/FLUIDS

After an activity – especially one that was intense – proper nutrition accelerates your recovery and better prepares you for your next physical challenge. The idea is to replenish your depleted glycogen stores and to expedite the recovery process as soon as possible after you train or compete.

Following an activity, it's best to consume foods that are high in carbohydrates with a high GI. These foods will help to restore your muscle glycogen in the quickest fashion. Foods with a relatively high GI include sports drinks, bananas, watermelons, raisins, rice cakes, cereals, pretzels, table sugar, white rice, baked potatoes, white bread, rye bread, bagels, pancakes and waffles.

Because appetite is suppressed immediately after intense efforts, it may be more practical for you to initially consume fluids rather than solid food or a meal. Cold fluids also help to cool the body. Commercial sports drinks can be excellent post-activity fluids. In terms of recovery, there are two important components of a sports drink: carbohydrates and electrolytes (sodium and potassium). Since all sports drinks are different, you should read the nutrition facts labels to be sure of their exact contents. As an example, 12 ounces of Gatorade® Energy Drink (The Gatorade Company) has 78 grams of carbohydrates which provide 312 calories; the same amount of Gatorade® Thirst Quencher contains 21 grams of carbohydrates which provide 84 calories. Both products have adequate amounts of electrolytes and a high GI but vastly different levels of carbohydrates and calories.

According to Nancy Clark, M. S., R. D. – an internationally known sports nutritionist and author – you should consume 0.5 grams of carbohydrates per pound of your bodyweight (g/lb) within two hours of completing an intense activity. This should be repeated again within the next two hours. For instance, an individual who weighs 180 pounds needs to ingest about 90 grams of carbohydrates – or 360 calories of carbohydrates – within two hours after an intense activity and another 90 grams of carbohydrates during the next two hours [0.5 g/lb x 180 lb].

There's some evidence to suggest that combining the carbohydrates with a small amount of protein can expedite recovery by improving the rate at which the glycogen stores are replenished. However, it appears that simply increasing the quantity of post-activity carbohydrates will have the same results. Nonetheless, consuming a small amount of protein following an intense activity may aid in the repair of muscle tissue.

Finally, it's also important to rehydrate after an activity. You should consume about 16 ounces of water for every pound of bodyweight that you lose during your training.

NUTRITIONAL SUPPLEMENTS

Skillful promoters regularly tout nutritional supplements – including protein, vitamins and minerals – with almost supernatural powers, having the ability to do practically everything imaginable. Individuals are frequently tempted, teased and seduced by their brilliant promises to "lose flab," "gain muscle," "get stronger" and "improve performance." Because of this, many people don't give a second thought to spending large sums of their money on a never-ending parade of nutritional supplements. Unfortunately, most of the claims concerning nutritional supplements are purely speculative and anecdotal with little or no scientific or medical basis.

Protein Supplements

Many active individuals think that they need to take protein supplements in order to increase their muscular strength and lean-body mass. A number of studies have shown that the protein needs of active individuals are higher than those of their inactive counterparts. But these needs have been drastically exaggerated and overrated by health-food manufacturers and promoters.

The fact of the matter is that individuals who consume adequate calories generally obtain sufficient protein. Recall that your caloric requirements are determined by several factors including your size and level of activity. Larger, more active individuals require and consume more calories than the average person. With these additional calories comes additional protein. In other words, the increased protein need is met by an increased caloric intake.

For adults, the RDA for protein is 0.8 grams per kilogram of bodyweight per day (g/kg/day). Assuming a sufficient caloric intake, 1.2 - 2.0 g/kg/day (about 1.5 - 2.5 times the RDA for adults) is present in any mixed diet that contains 15% of its calories as protein. Recall the 180-pound individual in the ongoing example who must consume 3,780 cal/day to maintain his bodyweight. If 15% of these calories came from protein, he'd receive 567 calories from protein or 141.75 grams [567 cal ÷ 4 cal/g]. Based upon the RDA of 0.8 g/kg/day, this individual would be consuming enough protein to meet the daily needs of a man who weighs nearly 390 pounds [141.75 g/day ÷ 0.8g/kg/day x 2.2 lb/kg = 389.81 lb]. This amount of protein is actually about 1.73 g/kg/day – or more than 2.15 times the RDA. And remember, this is without him making any effort to consume extra protein. So even if the requirement for active individuals may be greater, it's likely that they're already getting enough protein to ensure proper levels. If you're concerned that you aren't getting enough protein in your diet, you can obtain sufficient amounts by simply consuming more foods that are high in protein.

While on the subject, understand that an excessive intake of protein carries the potential for numerous unwanted side effects. An intake of protein that's in excess of the needs for growth, maintenance and repair of tissue is either stored as fat or excreted in the urine. When excessive protein is urinated, it places a heavy burden on the liver and kidneys and may damage those organs. An excessive intake of protein also increases the risk of dehydration which, in turn, increases the risk of developing a heat-related disorder such as heat exhaustion, heat stroke or heat cramps. Other potential side effects from a high intake of protein include an excessive loss of calcium in the urine, diarrhea, cramping and gastrointestinal upset.

Vitamin and Mineral Supplements

Many individuals believe that their foods don't supply sufficient micronutrients and, therefore, they take vitamin and mineral supplements. There's no unbiased, scientific evidence to suggest that those who consume a balanced diet need vitamin and mineral supplementation in excess of the RDA; likewise, there's no unbiased, scientific evidence to suggest that an increased consumption of vitamins and minerals improves performance. Recall that active individuals typically require and consume more calories than the average person. With these additional calories come additional vitamins and minerals. In truth, even a marginal diet provides adequate micronutrients. Understand, too, that your liver is a storehouse for vitamins and minerals. This organ can quickly compensate for a temporary dietary shortfall by releasing its stored micronutrients as needed and then replenishing its reservoirs when the opportunity arises.

That being said, vitamin and mineral supplements may be needed by those who don't consume adequate diets. For example, a multi-vitamin and -mineral supplement may be warranted for vegetarians and women who are pregnant or lactating. Supplementation may also be appropriate for individuals who restrict their caloric intakes because their sports have weight classifications (such as competitive weightlifting and judo). Since women are at an increased risk for iron and calcium deficiency, supplementation may be justified for those two minerals. Finally, a folate (folic acid) supplement may be warranted for women of childbearing age. (Professional advice concerning nutritional supplementation should be sought from a competent physician or registered dietitian.)

When taken in reasonable doses, vitamins and minerals pose no health or safety risks. The American Dietetic Association – the largest and most established organization devoted to both practice and research in nutrition – reports that megadoses of vitamins and minerals pose a risk of toxicity that can create adverse side effects and may lead to serious medical complications. When taken in megadoses – any dose greater than 10 times the RDA – vitamins and minerals that are in excess of those needed function as free-floating drugs. Like all drugs, high doses of vitamins and minerals have the potential for adverse side effects.

Of greatest concern is excessive intake of the fat-soluble vitamins – particularly vitamins A and D – which can be extremely toxic and may produce undesirable side effects. Consuming large doses of vitamin A can result in decalcification of bones (resulting in fragile bones), an increased susceptibility to disease, enlargements of the liver and spleen, muscle and joint soreness, vomiting, cessation of menstruation (amenorrhea), loss of appetite, loss of hair, irritability, double vision, skin rashes, headaches, nausea, drowsiness and diarrhea. Consuming large doses of vitamin D can result in nausea, loss of hair, loss of weight, vomiting, decalcification of bones, drowsiness, diarrhea, headaches, hypertension, elevated cholesterol and loss of appetite.

Excessive amounts of the B vitamins and vitamin C are generally excreted in the urine (which prompts many authorities to suggest that supplementation with water-soluble vitamins leaves a person with nothing more than expensive urine). This action places an inordinate amount of stress on the liver and kidneys. Though mainly excreted, excessive amounts of water-soluble vitamins may still have toxic effects. For example, an excessive intake of vitamin C can result in gout, kidney stones, diarrhea, bladder irritation, intestinal problems, destruction of red blood cells, nausea, stomach cramps, an increase in plasma cholesterol, ulceration of the gastric wall and leaching of calcium from bones.

FOOD FOR THOUGHT

As long as you consume a variety of foods that provide adequate calories and nutrients, there's no need for you to take nutritional supplements. By investing your money in high-quality foods instead of purchasing expensive nutritional supplements, you'll achieve greater success in maximizing your physical potential in a much safer manner. Remember, there are no shortcuts on the road to proper nutrition.

19
WATCHING YOUR WEIGHT

Managing your weight – that is, gaining, losing or maintaining it – is simply a matter of arithmetic and primarily a function of two variables: caloric consumption and caloric expenditure. If you consume more calories than you expend, you've produced a caloric profit and will gain weight; if you expend more calories than you consume, you've produced a caloric deficit and will lose weight; and lastly, if you consume the same amount of calories that you expend, you've produced a caloric balance and will not affect any change in your bodyweight.

A CLOSER LOOK

Despite its conceptual simplicity, a closer look should be taken at weight management. Specifically, it's worthwhile to examine gaining and losing weight in greater detail.

Gaining Weight

Some people would look and feel better if they increased their bodyweight. The potential to gain weight is determined by a number of things, the most important of which is a person's inherited characteristics. An individual whose ancestors had ectomorphic tendencies – that is, lean features with little in the way of muscular size – has the genetic destiny for that type of physique. This doesn't mean that a person with those inherited characteristics – who would be categorized as an "ectomorph" – is incapable of gaining weight. But it will be difficult for those who have a high degree of ectomorphy to achieve a significant increase in their bodyweight.

The primary goal of gaining weight is to increase lean-body (or muscle) mass. One pound of muscle has about 2,500 calories. Therefore, if you consume 250 calories per day (cal/day) above your caloric needs – a 250-calorie profit – it will take you 10 days to gain one pound of lean-body mass [2,500 cal ÷ 250 cal/day = 10 days]. So if you require 3,000 cal/day to maintain your bodyweight, you must consume 3,250 cal/day – 250 calories above your need – to gain one pound of lean-body mass in 10 days. (An equation for estimating your caloric needs is given in Chapter 18.)

The daily caloric profit shouldn't be more than about 350 - 700 calories above the normal daily needs which is about 1 - 2 pounds per week. If the weight gain is more than about 1% of your bodyweight per week, it's likely that some of it was due to an increase of body fat rather than lean-body mass. However, if the weight gain is less than about 1% of your bodyweight per week and is the result of a demanding strength-training program in conjunction with a moderate increase in caloric consumtion, then it will probably be in the form of increased lean-body mass.

Gaining weight requires total nutritional dedication for seven days a week. Additional calories must be consumed daily on a regular basis until the desired gain in weight is achieved. The best way for the body to absorb food is when it's divided into several regular-sized meals intermingled with a few snacks. The body doesn't absorb one or two large meals as well – most of these calories are simply jammed through the digestive system. When consuming a large number of calories at one time, some of them will be diverted to fat deposits because of the sudden demand on the metabolic pathways. (This has been referred to as "nutrient overload.")

Besides what has been discussed, here are some additional tips for gaining weight:

- Set short-term goals that are realistic
- Keep a food/activity log or diary
- Eat at least three meals per day

- Eat at least three nutritious snacks per day
- Consume foods that are high in calories (but not high in fat)
- Eat dense fruit (such as bananas, pineapples and raisins)
- Eat dense vegetables (such as peas, corn and carrots)
- Drink juice and milk
- Increase the size of portions

Losing Weight

Some people would look and feel better if they decreased their bodyweight. Similar to gaining weight, the potential to lose weight is primarily determined by a person's inherited characteristics. An individual whose ancestors had endomorphic tendencies – that is, round features with little in the way of muscular definition – has the genetic destiny for that type of physique. This doesn't mean that a person with those inherited characteristics – who would be categorized as an "endomorph" – is incapable of losing weight. But it will be difficult for those who have a high degree of endomorphy to achieve a significant decrease in their bodyweight.

Understand that the numbers on height/weight charts and bathroom scales are poor indicators of whether or not someone should lose weight. The need for weight loss should be determined by body composition rather than bodyweight, especially in the case of an active individual. Think about it: Two people could be same height and weight but have different body compositions. For example, one might have 15% body fat and the other 30% body fat. If this was the case, then only one person might need to lose weight – the one with the higher percentage of body fat.

The primary goal of losing weight is to decrease body fat. One pound of fat has about 3,500 calories. As such, if you consume 250 cal/day below your caloric needs – a 250-calorie deficit – it will take you 14 days to lose one pound of fat [3,500 cal ÷ 250 cal/day = 14 days]. So if you require 3,000 cal/day to maintain your bodyweight, you must consume 2,750 cal/day – 250 calories below your need – to lose one pound of fat in 14 days. (An equation for estimating your caloric needs is given in Chapter 18.)

Actually, a caloric deficit can be achieved by decreasing caloric consumption, increasing caloric expenditure (through additional activity) or a combination of the two. In fact, most authorities agree that proper weight loss should be a blend of consuming less calories and expending more calories. For instance, you can obtain a 250-calorie deficit by consuming 125 less calories and using 125 more calories.

The daily caloric deficit shouldn't be more than about 500 - 1000 calories below the normal daily needs which is about 1 - 2 pounds per week. If the weight loss is more than about 1% of your bodyweight per week, it's likely that some of it was due to a decrease of lean-body mass and/or water rather than body fat. However, if the weight loss is less than about 1% of your bodyweight per week and is the result of a rigorous training program in conjunction with a moderate decrease in caloric consumption, then it will probably be in the form of decreased body fat.

Losing weight must be a carefully planned activity. Skipping meals – or all-out starvation – isn't a desirable method of weight loss since sufficient calories are still needed to fuel an active lifestyle. Oddly enough, losing weight should be done in a fashion similar to that of gaining weight: Frequent – but smaller – meals should be consumed that are spread out over the course of the day. Doing this will suppress the appetite. It's also a good idea to drink plenty of water before, during and after meals. This creates a feeling of fullness without providing any calories.

Besides what has been discussed, here are some additional tips for losing weight:

- Set short-term goals that are realistic
- Keep a food/activity log or diary
- Read the nutrition facts labels
- Eat a moderate amount of sugars
- Eat foods that are low in fat
- Reduce the intake of saturated fats
- Eat more fruits and vegetables
- Chew your food slowly
- Decrease the size of portions

FAD DIETS

Make no mistake about it: Dieting is a multi-billion dollar business. As the term suggests,

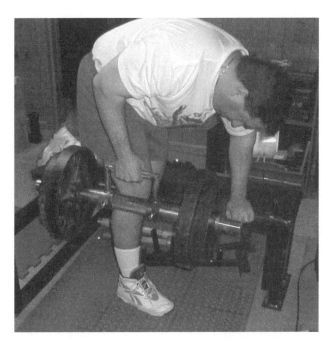

Photo 19-1: The best way to produce a caloric deficit to lose fat is through a combination of exercising more and eating less.

"fad" diets – like "fad" fashions – are those that are trendy for a while and then fade away only to resurface at some point in the future (sometimes with a new name). Fad diets have several things in common. First, they promise quick results – specifically, a rapid loss of weight. Second, they severely restrict one or more food groups or macronutrients. Third, they make big promises but offer little proof.

An endless stream of fad diets has been popular at one time or another. A partial list includes the Abs Diet, Algoxyll Diet, Ayurvedic Diet, Bikini Diet, Blood Type Diet, Body Type Diet, Brain Chemistry Diet, Burn Rate Diet, Cabbage Soup Diet, Carbohydrate Addict's Diet, Detox Diet, Fit for Life Diet, Grapefruit Diet, Hollywood 48-Hour Miracle Diet, Ice Cream Diet, Immune Power Diet, LA Diet, Liver Cleansing Diet, Mediterranean Diet, Metabolic Typing Diet, New Beverly Hills Diet, No-Grain Diet, Omega Diet, Origin Diet, Paleo Diet, Peanut Butter Diet, Pritikin Diet, Protein Power Diet, RealAge Diet, Resolution Diet, Scarsdale Diet, Slim Forever Diet, Southampton Diet, South Beach Diet, Starch Blocker Diet, Stillman Diet, Sugar Buster's Diet, 30-Day Low-Carb Diet, Three-Day Diet, Tri-Color Diet and Warrior Diet. But perhaps the two most popular diets of all time are the Atkins Diet and the Zone Diet.

The Atkins Diet

Promoted by Dr. Robert Atkins, this diet calls for a food intake that's low in carbohydrates and high in protein and fats. Dr Atkins endorsed the diet for more than 30 years until his death in April 2003 (from head injuries that were sustained in a fall on an icy sidewalk in New York City). Historically, diets seem to cycle in to and out of popularity and the Atkins Diet is no exception. Recently, the Atkins Diet has become fashionable again for two main reasons: (1) an article that was published in *The New York Times Magazine* by Gary Taubes and (2) the results of two independent studies that were published in the same issue of the *New England Journal of Medicine*.

In his article, Taubes enthusiastically endorsed the Akins Diet. However, many individuals in the scientific and medical communities responded to the article with quick and blistering rebuttals. Several who were quoted in the article claimed that Taubes had taken their words out of context or "tricked [them] all" into supporting the Atkins Diet; others claimed that he either disregarded or distorted their comments and provided information that was "incredibly misleading." One said that "[Taubes] ignored research that didn't agree with his conclusions." The shadow of doubt that this cast over his credibility renders the content of his article worthless.

The two studies that were published in a prestigious medical journal suggested that the Atkins Diet is more beneficial than previously thought. In both studies, for example, subjects who used a low-carbohydrate diet increased their high-density lipoproteins (the "good cholesterol") and decreased their triglycerides more than subjects who used a low-fat diet. (Elevated levels of triglycerides are associated with a greater risk of heart disease.)

Because this information is as surprising as it is tantalizing, the two studies demand greater scrutiny. Consider the following:

• Both studies had very high dropout rates. Of the 195 subjects in the beginning of the studies, only 116 completed the programs – a dropout rate of about 40.5%.

• Both of these studies involved obese and severely obese subjects, the results of which may not be relevant to other populations.

- Both studies were short-term (one was six months and the other one year).

- Technically, only one of the studies specifically used the Atkins Diet (the year-long study). In the other study, the subjects used a "carbohydrate-restricted (low-carbohydrate) diet" which certainly resembles the Atkins Diet but the term "Atkins Diet" wasn't mentioned or discussed by the researchers.

- Both studies involved very minimal supervision of the subjects which may have had an enormous impact on the results. For example, subjects in the six-month study received dietary instruction but it was up to them to follow the guidelines. In this study, the subjects in the low-carbohydrate group were told to "restrict carbohydrate intake to 30 [grams] per day or less"; the subjects in the low-fat group were told to restrict their calories so that it was "sufficient to create a deficit of 500 calories per day." In the year-long study, subjects who used the low-carbohydrate diet were given a copy of *Dr. Atkins' New Diet Revolution* and were told to "read the book and follow the diet as described"; subjects who used the low-fat diet were given a copy of *The LEARN Program for Weight Management* and told to "read the manual and follow the program as described." The gross lack of supervision raises a specter of uncertainty as to how closely the subjects followed their assigned protocols or even if they followed them at all.

- In the six-month study, data for the caloric intakes and the percentages of carbohydrates, protein and fats that were consumed per day by the subjects were based upon their "dietary recall." Perhaps even more astonishing, *no data whatsoever* were provided as to the caloric intakes and the percentages of carbohydrates, protein and fats that were consumed by the subjects throughout the course of the one-year study. Neither of the two studies made any mention of the caloric expenditures of the subjects. It's quite possible that a number of the subjects participated in some type of activity that expedited their weight loss. Without having accurate data or controlling for caloric in-

take/expenditure and macronutrient consumption, the effectiveness of two diets can't be compared. Indeed, who knows what the subjects actually consumed? These uncontrolled and unknown variables contaminate the scientific purity of the studies and make any results and conclusions highly suspect.

- Equally dubious is the fact that many of the analyses that were made by the researchers included data from *all of the subjects*. For the subjects who dropped out of the studies – a whopping 40.5% of the original subjects – their baseline values or last observed values were "carried forward." It's difficult to determine how the inclusion of data from individuals who didn't complete the studies might have influenced the results and conclusions of the research.

- Assuming for the moment that the caloric intake of the subjects in the six-month study is accurate, the group who used the low-carbohydrate diet consumed an average of 189 less calories per day than the group who used the low-fat diet. This may not seem significant but done daily over the course of six months (182 days), it amounts to a difference of nearly 10 pounds. In other words, the greater loss of weight that was experienced by the subjects who used the low-carbohydrate diet may have been the result of consuming fewer calories, not fewer carbohydrates.

- In the six-month study, the subjects who used the low-carbohydrate diet decreased their weight and triglycerides more than the subjects who used the low-fat diet. However, the authors noted that "it is unclear whether these benefits of a carbohydrate-restricted diet extend beyond six months."

- In the one-year study, the subjects who used the Atkins Diet lost more weight than the subjects who used the high-carbohydrate diet for the first six months. However, the subjects who used the Atkins Diet began regaining weight after six months and eventually regained more weight than the subjects on the high-carbohydrate diet. By the end of the year, there were no significant differences in weight loss between the groups.

- In the one-year study, the researchers noted

that "long-term adherence to the low-carbo-hydrate Atkins diet may be difficult."

Be aware that the Atkins Diet has several caveats. First, most of the initial weight loss is water, not fat. Second, it's very structured and strict with limited food choices thereby making it difficult to maintain. Third, any diet that's based upon a low intake of carbohydrates is also low in fruits, vegetables and whole-grain products. Four, the diet is high in meat, butter, cheese, saturated fat and other artery cloggers which is very unhealthy. Five, the long-term safety and effectiveness of the diet are unknown.

A final point: One of the foundations of the Atkins Diet is that high-glycemic foods increase blood-insulin levels which lowers blood glucose (sugar). While this is true, there's no evidence that this hormonal reaction causes an individual to gain weight. Understand that any weight loss that's produced by the Atkins Diet is because of a reduction in the amount of calories, not a re-duction in the amount of carbohydrates. You can lose weight with any diet as long as the calories that you consume are less than the calories that you need.

The Zone Diet

Invented and promoted by Dr. Barry Sears, the Zone Diet calls for a food intake that consists of 40% carbohydrates, 30% protein and 30% fat. There's very little scientific evidence that the Zone Diet is more effective than other diets. In one study, subjects were randomly assigned to one of two diets that provided 1,200 calories per day. One group followed the Zone Diet and the other a "traditional" diet that consisted of 65% carbo-hydrates, 15% protein and 25% fat. After six weeks, both groups had similar losses of bodyweight and body fat. The fact of the matter is that any weight loss experienced from the Zone Diet – or any other diet, for that matter – is the result of caloric restriction.

With that said, there are a number of con-cerns with the Zone Diet. For one thing, follow-ing the diet doesn't allow for the intake of a vari-ety of foods that are required to meet nutritional needs. Rather, the Zone Diet – similar to the Atkins Diet – calls for the consumption of a high amount of protein and fats. To achieve this, you must decrease your intake of carbohydrates. Doing so restricts the intake of healthy foods – such as fruits, vegetables and whole-grain products – which may lead to vitamin and mineral deficien-cies. Since fewer carbohydrates are available as a source of energy, you'll also fatigue more quickly during physical activities.

More importantly, however, the Zone Diet (and Atkins Diet) poses significant health risks. The National Research Council recommends against consuming protein in amounts greater than twice the Recommended Dietary Allowance because high intakes are associated with certain cancers and heart disease. A high intake of fat is also associated with heart disease. Consider this: In the aforementioned study, the group that used the "traditional" diet had a decrease in triglyc-erides while the group that used the Zone Diet had an increase. In addition, a high intake of protein increases the levels of uric acid which may cause gout in those who are susceptible. Excreting an excessive amount of protein stresses the liver and kidneys. There are additional con-cerns as well.

THE BOTTOM LINE

Whether you're interested in gaining, los-ing or maintaining your bodyweight, your best bet is to stick to the basics. If you want to gain weight (lean-body mass), you must consume more calories than you expend; if you want to lose weight (fat), you must expend more calories than you consume; and if you want to maintain your weight, you must consume the same amount of calories that you expend. Finally, keep in mind that the best way to produce a caloric deficit to lose fat is through a combination of exercising more and eating less.

20

AT-HOME Q&A

This final chapter examines a number of frequently asked questions concerning your at-home training. No doubt, many of you have the same or similar questions.

Q: How do I know if I'm overtraining?

A: Overtraining is a result of overstressing your body. Generally speaking, the excessive stress is produced by excessive activity. Symptoms of overtraining include chronic fatigue, appetite disorders, insomnia, depression, anger, substantial weight loss or gain, prolonged muscular soreness, anemia and an elevated resting heart rate.

The most obvious indicator of overtraining, however, is a lack of progress in your workouts. You can identify a lack of progress by keeping accurate records of your performances.

The best cure for overtraining is to obtain sufficient rest in order to allow your body the opportunity to recover. This may necessitate reducing the volume of activity that you perform (in terms of workouts, exercises and/or sets). Taking some time off periodically from your workouts also helps to avoid overtraining.

Q: How can I change my body type?

A: Unfortunately, you cannot change your body type to any significant degree. There are three main body types: endomorph, mesomorph and ectomorph.

Endomorphs are characterized by soft, round physiques. They have high percentages of body fat and very little muscle tone. Mesomorphs are typified by heavily muscled physiques. They have athletic builds with broad shoulders, large chests and slender waists. Finally, ectomorphs are characterized by lean, slender physiques. They have low percentages of body fat but also little in the way of muscular size.

Relatively few people can be classified as being purely one body type or another. Although people have a tendency toward one body type, most are a combination of two types. For example, an individual who has a slender physique, a low percentage of body fat and a high degree of muscular development would be characterized as an ecto-mesomorph; an individual who has a round physique, a high percentage of body fat and a high degree of muscular development

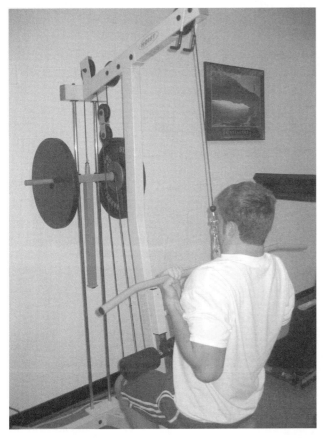

Photo 20-1: Taking some time off periodically from your workouts helps to avoid overtraining.

would be characterized as an endo-mesomorph.

Q: Is the Body-Mass Index a valid indicator of being overweight or obese?

A: The Body-Mass Index (or BMI) is simply a ratio of someone's height to weight. It has been used as a quick and handy way to estimate if a person is overweight (or underweight). But keep in mind that the BMI is just that: an *estimate*. Understand that individuals can have a high BMI yet they may not need to lose any weight. Consider this example: An individual who is 5'10" and weighs 209 pounds has a BMI of more than 29.9 which is categorized as obese. But this happens to be the height and weight of Emmitt Smith who has rushed for more yards than any running back in the history of the National Football League. A quick glance at this future Hall of Famer would reveal that he's not anywhere near being obese. In fact, his percentage of body fat is undoubtedly in the single digits. So, the BMI can certainly be used to estimate if someone needs to lose (or gain) weight but body composition – specifically, the percentage of body fat – is a much more valid indicator.

Q: Does stretching prior to a physical activity reduce the risk of injury?

A: There's very little research that has investigated the effects of pre-exercise/activity stretching on the risk of injury. But two studies that involved a total of 2,630 military recruits (men aged 17 - 35) who were going through basic training found that stretching prior to an activity reduced the risk of injury by 5% (which wasn't statistically significant). Over the same period of time, the expected risk of injury was 20%. This suggests that a 5% reduction in the risk of injury would translate into a reduction in absolute risk by a mere 1%. Stretching would seem to be most beneficial when done prior to dynamic, short-duration activities that involve rapid muscular contractions such as sprinting.

Q: Does walking a mile use the same number of calories as running a mile?

A: The American College of Sports Medicine offers equations for determining oxygen consumption and caloric expenditure during walking and running. Based upon these equations, a 200-pound man who walks one mile in 20 minutes on a level surface will utilize roughly 5.25 calories per minute (cal/min). Over the course of his 20-minute walk, his total caloric usage would be about 105.0 calories [5.25 cal/min x 20 min]. If that same individual ran one mile in 10 minutes on a level surface, he'd use about 16.22 cal/min. During his 10-minute effort, his total caloric expenditure would be about 162.2 calories [16.22 cal/min x 10 min]. So, running a mile utilized significantly more calories than walking a mile [162.2 cal compared to 105.0 cal]. This is true despite the fact that the duration of walking was twice as long as that of running [20 min compared to 10 min].

Q: Are there differences in the energy requirements between running outdoors on a road and running indoors on a treadmill?

A: Assuming that "running outdoors on a road" is done in a relatively calm environment (meaning the wind doesn't offer any substantial amount of air resistance), not really. In one study, eight subjects (who were runners) ran on a track and a treadmill at three different speeds: 6.7, 7.8 and 9.7 miles per hour. The researchers found that, statistically, there were no significant differences in the energy requirements between running on a track and a treadmill. So, you can still simulate an outdoor effort – and obtain other health and fitness benefits – by running on a treadmill in the comfort of your home.

Q: How accurately does a treadmill estimate caloric expenditure?

A: The numbers given on the console of a treadmill can be quite accurate. The accuracy of the caloric expenditure or any other data that are displayed on the console of a treadmill – or any other cardio machine – depends upon the accuracy of the equations that are programmed into a computer chip. And, of course, you must enter your correct bodyweight for the caloric expenditure to be accurate.

Q: Is it true that a person doesn't start using fat as an energy source until after 20 minutes of exercise?

A: The main source of energy that's used during an activity depends upon the level of effort, not the time of the effort. At rest, your body primarily uses fat as an energy source. As the level of effort increases, there's a greater reliance on carbohydrates to provide energy. So, you don't have to exercise for 20 minutes before using fat as a source of energy. In fact, as you read this book, your body is primarily using fat as an energy source. Besides, it's ridiculous to think that the body automatically switches to fat as an energy source at exactly the 20-minute mark.

Q: Is low-intensity exercise better than high-intensity exercise for fat/weight loss?

A: As just noted, training with a relatively low level of intensity uses a greater percentage of fat; training with a relatively high level of intensity uses a greater percentage of carbohydrates. These physiological facts have led to the mistaken belief that low-intensity activity is better than high-intensity activity when it comes to using fat as well as losing weight. Furthermore, this misconception has spawned the hyped-up notion that people should exercise within their "fat-burning zones."

In truth, even though a greater *percentage* of fat calories are used during low-intensity activity, a greater *number* of fat calories (and *total* calories) are used during high-intensity activity. In one study, a group of subjects walked on a treadmill at an average speed of 3.8 miles per hour (mph) for 30 minutes. In this instance, the subjects used an average of 240 calories of which 59% [144] were from carbohydrates and 41% [96] were from fat. As part of the study, the same group also ran on a treadmill at an average speed of 6.5 mph for 30 minutes. At this relatively higher level of intensity, the subjects used an average of 450 calories of which 76% [342] were from carbohydrates and 24% [108] were from fat. In other words, training with a higher level of intensity resulted in a greater total caloric expenditure than training with a lower level of intensity [450 calories compared to 240] and also used a greater number of calories from fat in the same length of time [108 calories compared to 96].

Researchers in the area of exercise and weight management generally agree that it probably doesn't matter whether fat or carbohydrates are used while training in order to lose fat/weight. The main determinant of fat/weight loss is calories, not composition. As long as it's physically and psychologically tolerable, exercising with a high level of intensity is preferable.

Q: If I do aerobic training and strength training in the same workout, which one should I do first?

A: If your main goal is increasing your muscular strength, then strength training should be done before aerobic training; if your main goal is increasing your aerobic fitness, then aerobic training should be done before strength training.

But what if your main goal is improving your overall fitness? Well, research indicates that better results are obtained when aerobic training is performed before strength training. In one study, subjects did strength training, rested for 5 minutes and then did aerobic training (pedaling for 20 minutes on a stationary cycle). During a subsequent workout, the same subjects did the same activities but in reverse sequence: They did aerobic training, rested for 5 minutes and then did strength training. When they did strength training after aerobic training, their strength performance was 1% worse than when they did strength training before aerobic training; when they did aerobic training after strength training, their aerobic performance was 8% worse than when they did aerobic training before strength training. If both activities are to be done in the same workout, then, aerobic training has less of an impact on strength training than strength training has on aerobic training.

Q: How do I choose a personal trainer?

A: No doubt, some people who train in their homes will consider hiring a personal trainer on either a short- or long-term basis. Among other things, the right trainer can help motivate and educate you to achieve your goals. Here's a checklist of some areas to take into account when hiring a trainer:

- What's the background/experience of the trainer?
- Did the trainer earn a college degree in a related field (such as exercise physiology, exercise science, kinesiology or physical education)?
- Has the trainer made an effort for continued education by attending conferences/seminars and reading current research in scientific pub-

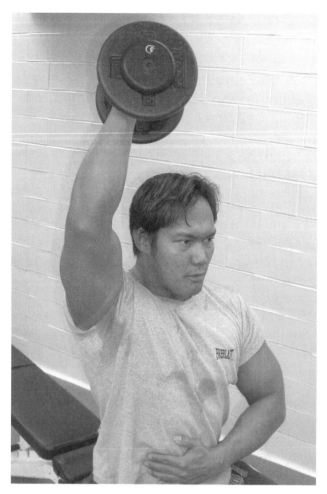

there discounted "packages" for purchasing chunks of time)?

- Can the trainer provide several references of past and current clients?

One last point: Understand that a trainer might not have a college degree in a related field – or even a certification – but can make up for this lack of formal instruction with knowledge learned from applicable experiences and self-education.

Q: Is there a certain way that I should breathe when I lift weights?

A: It's important for you to breath properly when you perform an activity such as strength training – especially during intense efforts. Holding your breath during exertion creates an elevated pressure in your abdominal and thoracic cavities. The elevated pressure interferes with the return of blood to your heart. This may deprive your brain of blood and can cause you to lose consciousness.

To emphasize correct breathing, exhale when you raise the resistance and inhale when you lower it. Or simply remember EOE – Exhale On Effort. As it turns out, inhaling and exhaling naturally usually results in correct breathing.

Q: If I stop lifting weights my muscles will turn to fat, right?

A: It's a common misconception that muscle can turn into fat. In truth, muscle cannot be changed into fat – or vice versa – any more than gold can be changed into lead. Your muscle tissue consists of special contractile proteins that allow movement to occur. Muscle tissue is about 70% water, 22% protein and 7% fat. (The remaining 1% or so includes inorganic salts such as calcium, potassium and sodium.) Conversely, your fatty tissue is composed of spherical cells that are specifically designed to store fat. Fatty tissue is about 22% water, 6% protein and 72% fat. Since muscle and fat are two different and distinct types of biological tissue, a muscle cannot turn into fat if you stop lifting weights. Similarly, lift-

lications (*not* the fitness and "muscle" magazines on the newsstand)?

- Does the trainer have a credible certification from a nationally recognized organization?
- Does the trainer have a current certification in First Aid/CPR/AED?
- Does the trainer have liability insurance to protect against an unfortunate injury to you or damage to your property?
- Can the trainer adjust your training to meet your special needs?
- Is the trainer compatible with your psychological profile?
- What are the trainer's abilities to listen and communicate?
- Is the trainer professional, courteous and responsive?
- Is the trainer available when it's convenient for you?
- How much will you be charged for personal training and can you "pay as you go" (or are

ing weights – or doing any other type of physical activity – will not change your fat into muscle. The fact is that muscles hypertrophy (or become larger) from physical activity and muscles atrophy (or become smaller) from physical inactivity.

Q: Will lifting weights make me muscle-bound and inflexible?

A: First of all, achieving a heavily muscled physique is easier said than done. Everyone can increase their muscle mass (and strength) but the degree to which this is done is a function of an individual's genetics. Second, there's no correlation whatsoever between muscle mass and flexibility. While some people who are very muscular have poor flexibility, other people who are very muscular have outstanding flexibility. Consider John Grimek who was perhaps the most muscular man of his generation. He won the 1940 and 1941 AAU (Amateur Athletic Union) Mr. America, the 1946 AAU America's Most Muscular Physique and the 1948 Mr. Universe (where he beat the legendary Steve Reeves of Hercules fame). Grimek had a heavily muscled physique but was flexible enough to do a front split.

As noted in Chapter 5, a properly conducted strength-training program doesn't reduce flexibility. In fact, exercising throughout a full range of motion against a resistance will maintain – or even improve – flexibility. If you have residual fears about losing flexibility, you can perform a comprehensive stretching routine both before and after your strength-training workout. As an added measure, you can also stretch your muscles immediately after you complete each exercise. (Detailed information on designing a flexibility program is given in Chapter 3.)

Q: Don't I need to do any warm-up sets prior to a set in which I exercise to the point of muscular fatigue?

A: Just because you didn't do any warm-up sets doesn't mean that you aren't warmed up. From a physiological perspective, an adequate warm-up is one in which the core temperature

is increased by one degree. If you do a relatively high number of repetitions and lift the weight in a deliberate, controlled fashion without any explosive or jerking movements, then you'll actually warm-up as you do the exercise. Think about it: If you do a set of 10 repetitions with a speed of movement that's roughly six seconds per repetition, you'll have exercised your muscles for about one minute before you reach muscular fatigue. After one minute of exercising, there's little doubt that you'll be adequately warmed up and prepared – both physiologically and psychologically – to exercise to muscular fatigue.

An exception to this would be someone such as a competitive weightlifter who does low-repetition sets. In this case, one or more warm-up sets should be done prior to the low-repetition efforts to reduce the risk of injury.

Q: When I lift weights, is it better for me to increase the resistance or the repetitions?

A: Regardless of the program being implemented, one of the key tenets in strength training is that of progressive overload. In brief, your muscles must experience a workload that's in-

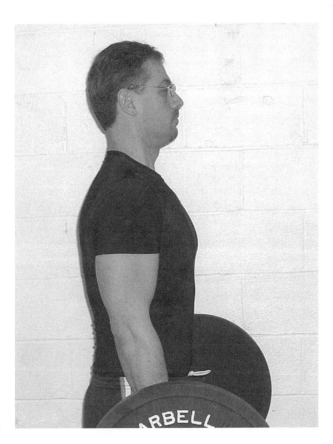

Photo 20-3: Everyone can increase their muscle mass (and strength) but the degree to which this is done is a fuction of an individual's genetics.

creased steadily and systematically throughout the course of your strength-training program. You can increase the workload two ways (in a subsequent workout): Use more resistance or do more repetitions. Either way, you've placed a "load" upon your muscles that's "over" what they're accustomed to using – thus the term "overload." There's one caveat, however: You can increase the repetitions that you do with a given weight as long as the duration of the set is kept within an anaerobic window of time (which is less than about two minutes).

Q: Do higher repetitions build muscular endurance instead of muscular strength?

A: It has been believed that doing higher repetitions (with a lighter weight) builds muscular endurance and doing lower repetitions (with a heavier weight) builds muscular strength. Actually, muscular endurance and muscular strength are directly related. If you increase your muscular endurance, you'll also increase your muscular strength. Here's an example: Suppose that your predicted one-repetition maximum (1-RM) in the bench press is 150 pounds and you can do 10 repetitions with 112.5 pounds (75% of 150). And after several months of strength training with higher repetitions – say, within a range of about 8 - 12 – suppose that you've progressed to the point where you can do 135 pounds for 10 repetitions. Given that you increased the amount of weight that you could lift for 10 repetitions in the bench press by 20% – from 112.5 to 135 pounds – it's likely that your 1-RM strength will now be greater than your previous 1-RM effort of 150 pounds. So even though you trained with higher repetitions, you increased your muscular strength.

By the way, it works the other way as well. If you increase your muscular strength, you'll also increase your muscular endurance. Here's why: As you get stronger, you need fewer muscle fibers to sustain a sub-maximal effort (muscular endurance). This also means that you have a greater reserve of muscle fibers available to extend the sub-maximal effort.

Q: Should I do higher repetitions to "tone" my muscles and lower repetitions to "bulk" them?

A: There's no scientific evidence that higher repetitions increase muscular definition ("tone")

and lower repetitions increase muscular size ("bulk"). In one study, there were no significant differences in muscular size (and strength) between a group that trained with sets of four repetitions and a group that trained with sets of 10 repetitions. In another study, there were no significant differences in muscular size between a group that trained with sets of 3 - 5 repetitions, a group that trained with sets of 13 - 15 repetitions and a group that trained with sets of 23 - 25 repetitions.

If you and another person perform the same program – that is, the same exercises as well as the same number of sets and repetitions – for a period of time, it's highly unlikely that you'll end up looking like physical clones of each other. People respond differently to strength training because each person – except for identical twins – is a unique genetic entity with a different genetic potential for achieving muscular size (and strength). Some people are predisposed toward developing heavily muscled physiques while others are predisposed toward developing highly defined physiques. Whether your sets consist of low repetitions or high repetitions, you're still going to develop according to your genetic (or inherited) blueprint – provided that you do your sets with similar levels of intensity.

Understand that your response to strength training isn't necessarily due to a particular program. Following the program of a successful bodybuilder doesn't mean that you'll develop the same level of muscular size; likewise, following the program of a successful weightlifter doesn't mean that you'll develop the same level of physical strength.

Q: Will lifting weights make women develop large muscles?

A: A popular misconception in strength training is the belief that women will develop large, unsightly muscles. Understand that increases in muscular strength are often accompanied by increases in muscular size. While this is true for men and women, the fact of the matter is that increases in muscular size are much less pronounced in women. Studies have shown that most women can achieve significant gains in their muscular strength without concomitant gains in their muscular size. One researcher, for example, found that a group of 47 women increased their strength in the leg press *by nearly 30%* after 10 weeks of exercising yet the largest increase in muscular size that was experienced by any of them was *less than one-quarter inch*. Clearly, strength training doesn't produce excessive muscular size in the majority of women.

There are several physiological reasons that prevent or minimize a woman's potential to significantly increase the size of their muscles. For instance, most women have low levels of testosterone. The low levels of this growth-promoting hormone restrict the degree to which they can increase their muscular size. In addition, women tend to inherit higher percentages of body fat than do men. This extra body fat tends to soften or mask the effects of strength training.

If you're wondering about female bodybuilders, they've inherited a greater potential to increase the size of their muscles than the average woman. Highly competitive female bodybuilders have developed large muscles because of their genetic potential – not simply because they lifted weights. Keep in mind, too, that female bodybuilders look much more muscular while posing on stage than they actually are in a relaxed state. While training for a competition, female bodybuilders have restricted their caloric intakes – often severely – thereby reducing their body fat and body fluids. Immediately prior to posing on stage, they've also "pumped" their muscles. This engorges their muscles with blood and makes them temporarily bigger. Finally, the stage lighting as well as their tans and clothing – and even the oil that's rubbed on their bodies – all contribute to making female bodybuilders appear as if they have much more muscular size than they really do.

Q: Will I respond differently if I do the bench press with a machine rather than a barbell?

A: Not really. In truth, any exercise that progressively applies a load on your muscles will stimulate improvements in muscular size and strength. The bench press – whether it's done with a machine or a barbell – addresses the same major muscles, namely the chest, anterior deltoids and triceps. Although balancing a barbell requires a greater involvement of synergistic muscles, it doesn't appear as if this results in a significantly greater response. Indeed, studies have shown that there are no significant differences in the development of strength when comparing groups who used free weights and groups who used machines.

The bottom line is that your muscles don't have eyes, brains or cognitive ability. Therefore, they cannot possibly know whether the source of resistance is a barbell, a machine or a cinder block. The sole factors that determine your response from strength training are your genetic profile and level of effort – not the equipment that you used. To quote Dan Riley, the Strength and Conditioning Coach of the Houston Texans who has spent more than 22 years in the National Football League, "The equipment used is not the key to maximum gains. It's how you use the equipment."

Q: Is the barbell squat the best exercise for training the lower body?

A: Everything else being equal, the best exercises for increasing muscular size and strength are those that involve the greatest amounts of muscle mass. Since the barbell squat addresses such an enormous amount of muscle mass – namely, the hips, upper legs and lower back – it qualifies as being a very good exercise for train-

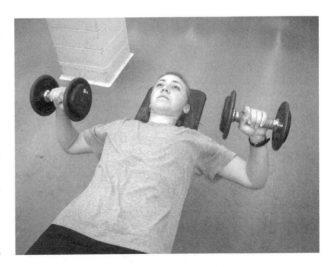

Photo 20-4: A popular miscenception in strength training is the belief that women will develop large, unsightly muscles.

ing the lower body. But the barbell squat has an inherent disadvantage in that many people – because of their body type and/or physical condition – cannot perform the exercise in manner that's orthopedically safe.

One orthopedic concern is the knee. In order to maintain your balance during the descending phase of the barbell squat, you must move your knees forward of your ankles (from a horizontal perspective). The farther the knee moves forward, the greater the stretch of the joint and the greater the shear (side-to-side) force in the patellar tendon. As the length of the legs increases, so does the distance that the knees move forward of the ankles. Therefore, someone with long legs is more prone to the shearing or "grinding" effect in the knees than someone with short legs.

A second area of orthopedic concern is the lower back. Squatting with a barbell on the shoulders compresses the spinal column which, in extreme cases, could result in a herniated or ruptured disc. Everything else being equal, someone with a long torso is subjected to higher compressive loads in the lower back than someone with a short torso.

A great exercise that you can do in your home that addresses the extensive musculature of your lower body without the inherent risk of injury to your knees and lower back is a squat with a stability ball. In this exercise, you have the freedom to position your lower legs so that there's minimal shear force in your knees and there's no spinal compression. (A detailed description of this exercise can be found in Chapter 6.)

Q: Why is it easier to do a lat pulldown with an underhand grip than an overhand grip?

A: Regardless of how you position your hands, just about any type of pulling movement for the torso – whether it's rowing, chinning or any pulling variation – targets the same muscles, namely your upper back (or "lats"), biceps and forearms. However, there are differences in the leverage that you receive from your musculoskeletal system based upon the grip that's used. Performing a lat pulldown with an underhand grip (your palms facing you) is more biomechanically efficient than doing a lat pulldown with an overhand grip (your palms away from you). With an underhand grip, the radius and ulna (the bones in your lower arm) run parallel to one another; with an overhand grip, the radius crosses over the ulna forming an "X". In this position, the bicep tendon gets wrapped around the lower portion of the radius, creating a biomechanical disadvantage and a loss in leverage.

Q: What's the best exercise for getting rid of the "spare tire" around my midsection?

A: The abdominal area probably gets more attention than any other bodypart. Many people perform countless repetitions of sit-ups, knee-ups and other abdominal exercises – sometimes more than once per day – with the belief that this will give them a highly prized set of "washboard abs."

Abdominal exercises certainly involve your abdominal muscles. But the exercises have little effect on the subcutaneous fat that resides over the abdominal muscles (and below your skin). The reason why you cannot selectively lose fat from an isolated area is that when you exercise, fat (and carbohydrate) stores are drawn from throughout your body as a source of fuel – not just from one specific area. So, you can do an endless amount of abdominal exercises but these Olympian efforts will not automatically trim your mid-section. In one study, researchers evaluated the effects of a 27-day sit-up program on the fat-cell diameter and body composition of 13 subjects. Over this four-week period, each subject performed a total of 5,004 sit-ups (with the legs bent at a 90-degree angle and no foot support). Fat biopsies from the abdominal, subscapular and gluteal sites revealed that the sit-up program reduced the fat-cell diameter at all three sites to a similar degree. In other words, exercising the abdominal muscles didn't preferentially affect the fat in the abdominal area more than the gluteal or subscapular areas.

You should treat your abdominals just like any other muscle. Once an activity for your abdominals exceeds about 70 seconds in duration, it becomes an increasingly greater test of aerobic (or muscular) endurance rather than muscular strength. Your abdominals can be targeted effectively in a time-efficient manner by

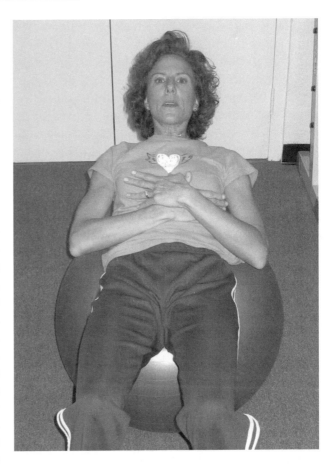

Photo 20-5: Your abdominals can be targeted effectively in a time-efficient manner by training to the point of muscular fatigue within about 10-12 repetitions (or about 60 - 70 seconds).

training them to the point of muscular fatigue within about 10 - 12 repetitions (or about 60 - 70 seconds).

Q: How can I make smaller progressions in resistance when using dumbbells?

A: If you don't have adjustable dumbbells, you can purchase them in smaller increments such as 7.5, 12.5, 17.5 and 22.5 pounds. If that option is prohibitive because of cost or space, you can buy magnetic add-on weights that can be secured to the ends of dumbbells. This allows you to make increases in resistance that are much more desirable. So instead of having to jump from 10- to 15-pounders – a 50% increase in resistance – you can create a pair of dumbbells that weigh 12.5 pounds. Some companies sell magnetic add-on weights that weigh as little as 1.25 pounds. These weights can be round or hex to match the shape of the dumbbells in your home gym. Here's one other inexpensive tip for you to make smaller progressions with dumbbells: You can wear ankle/wrist weights. If you use 20-pound dumbbells while wearing 2.5-pound weights on your wrists, it makes for 22.5 pounds of resistance.

Q: Is there anything that I can do to make increases that are smaller than 10-pound increments on my cable column?

A: While some cable columns offer a self-contained system of making smaller progressions (such as "drop-down" weights), others don't give you that luxury. Yet, it's important to be able to "micro-load" in smaller increments. Remember, making a 10-pound progression from 100 to 110 pounds is an increase of 10%; making a 10-pound progression from 20 to 30 pounds is an increase of 50%. So progressions should be thought of in relative terms, not absolute. Being able to make a smaller increase represents a more reasonable – and manageable – progression.

If your cable column doesn't allow you to make smaller progressions in the resistance, you can purchase saddle plates (or "add-on weights") that can be placed on the top plate of the weight

stack. Standard weights for saddle plates are 2.5 and 5 pounds. Another option is to purchase magnetic add-on weights that can be secured to the front of the weight stack. Or if you have plates for barbells, you can secure one of them to the weight stack by first inserting a selector pin through its hole and then into a selectorized plate. Actually, you can make a smaller progression in resistance by placing any light object of known weight on the top plate of the weight stack – as long as it won't fall off while you use the cable column.

Q: What's the earliest age that a youth can begin strength training?

A: Determining the earliest age that a youth can safely begin strength training is based upon skeletal development. Chronologically, a 13-year-old may have the skeleton of an 11-year-old; another 13-year-old may have the skeleton of a 15-year-old. These wide individual variations in physical maturation can make it difficult to establish a reasonably safe age at which a youth can begin strength training.

In terms of assessing physical readiness, it's important to consider the adolescent growth spurt – a period of accelerated increases in height and weight that occurs with the onset of adolescence. The age of onset and the duration of the spurt vary considerably from one individual to another. The average boy begins his adolescent growth spurt at about the age of 13; the average girl begins her adolescent growth spurt about two years earlier.

As you can see, there's no clear-cut borderline for determining when to begin strength training because each youth "ages" at a different rate. Nevertheless, most youths are physically mature enough to begin strength training at about the age of 13 or 14. Prior to that, youths can perform calisthenic-type exercises involving their bodyweight such as push-ups and crunches. They can also be introduced to strength training by exercising with "low-level" resistance bands/cords.

Q: How effective is it to do exercises on a stability ball?

A: In a recent study that involved eight physically active men, researchers examined the effects of performing isometric contractions under conditions that were unstable (sitting on a Swiss ball) and stable (sitting on a bench). Here's what they found: In the unstable condition, the force output during a leg extension was 70.5% less than in the stable condition. In other words,

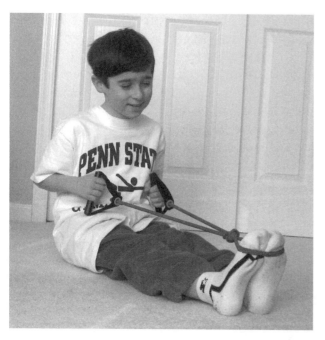

the force output while doing a leg extension on an unstable ball was only 29.5% of the force output while doing a leg extension on a stable bench. And in the unstable condition, the activation of the quadriceps during a leg extension was 44.3% less than in the stable condition. So, more instability correlated to less force production and less muscle activation.

Needless to say, this isn't desirable when it comes to strength training. That being said, exercising on stability balls can be used to provide variety to workouts.

Q: Is there anything wrong with eating an energy bar when I miss a meal?

A: First, keep in mind that use of the term "energy" can be misleading. Numerous products use the word "energy" in their names. This suggests that the product will improve your stamina or make you more energetic. In truth, calories provide you with energy and three nutrients provide you with calories: carbohydrates, protein and fat. In short, you get energy from food. Technically, then, a can of soda is an "energy drink," a hot dog is an "energy roll," a pad of butter is an "energy square," a slice of bacon is an "energy strip," a chocolate-chip cookie is an "energy disc" and an ice-cream sandwich is an "energy bar." That being said, there's nothing inherently "wrong" with most of the products that have been dubbed "energy bars." So, you can eat an energy bar – especially when it's more convenient for you because of time constraints. Just don't make a habit of eating energy bars rather than regular foods and meals. Remember, there's nothing wrong with energy bars . . . but there's nothing magical about them, either.

Q: Is it true that carbohydrates make you fat?

A: The truth is that eating too much and exercising too little make you fat. If anything, it's important for you to consume carbohydrates to fuel your athletic lifestyle. The primary function of carbohydrates is to supply you with energy – especially during intense exertions. The other two

---

Photo 20-6: Prior to the age of about 13 or 14, youths can be introduced to strength training by exercising with "low-level" resistance bands/cords.

macronutrients that are sources of energy – protein and fat – have major limitations for active individuals. Fat is an inefficient source of energy so it's preferred during low-intensity efforts when there's no need to be efficient; protein is actually a last resort since it's located in your muscles and if you're in a situation where you must rely on it as an energy source, then you're literally cannibalizing yourself. In short, eliminating carbohydrates from your diet will inhibit your stamina and endurance.

In addition, consuming too much protein and fat is associated with a greater risk of heart disease. And if you avoid carbohydrates, you also avoid foods with highly valuable nutrients such as fruits, vegetables and whole grains. This may lead to vitamin and mineral deficiencies. Clearly, carbohydrates are miscast villains.

Q: Is every carbohydrate the same?

A: All carbohydrates aren't created equal. A source of carbohydrates is a banana . . . but so is a soda. Carbohydrates that are more desirable include fruits, vegetables and whole grains; they're full of vitamins and fiber. Carbohydrates that are less desirable include processed foods such as cakes, cookies and muffins as well as soft drinks and candy; obviously, they're not as nutritious as healthier carbohydrates.

Q: What exactly are "net carbs"?

A: In response to carbohydrate paranoia, many manufacturers have been using the term "net carbs" (as well as "effective carbs" or "impact carbs") on the packaging of their food products (though not on the nutrition facts labels). The food industry calculates net carbs by taking the total grams of carbohydrates per serving and then subtracting the grams of fiber and sugar alcohols (which are neither sugar nor alcohol; rather, they're sweeteners).

Food manufacturers claim that because fiber isn't digested and sugar alcohols have a negligible effect on blood glucose, they "don't count." It's true that fiber passes through the digestive system largely intact and sugar alcohols (such as sorbitol and maltitol) have a minimum impact on blood glucose. But here's where the math gets fuzzy: Sugar alcohols have calories and, thus, "do count."

Understand that "net carbs" is an unscientific term that's calculated in a subjective way. Clearly, it was invented and implemented by the food industry to capitalize on the low-carb frenzy. At the present time, net carbs – and other popular terms that are used on product packaging such as "low-carb" – haven't been defined or even recognized by the Food and Drug Administration (which is why they don't appear on the nutrition facts label).

Q: Will creatine improve my athletic performance?

A: There are many anecdotal reports that creatine is effective but scientific research paints a different picture. Much of the research that has investigated creatine has been conducted in a laboratory. In this controlled setting, the best evidence for performance enhancement from the use of creatine is in repeated maximal, short-term sprints on a stationary bicycle. And even then, some studies have shown no improvements. Of the research that has been done outside a laboratory, very few studies have shown that creatine improves athletic performances in activities such as swimming and running. For example, two studies using a total of 52 elite male and female swimmers found that creatine didn't improve performance in a 100-meter swim; a study using 18 well-trained male runners showed that creatine produced significantly *slower* times in a 6,000-meter run.

While on the subject, keep in mind that the long-term effects of creatine supplementation are unknown. There's also a fear that many individuals typically exceed the recommended dosage – undoubtedly putting them at a greater risk for incurring adverse side effects. Of greatest concern is the potential for water retention, muscle cramping, dehydration/heat-related illness, muscle strains/dysfunction, gastrointestinal distress (such as an upset stomach, gastrointestinal pain, flatulence, nausea and vomiting) and liver and kidney dyfunction.

Based upon the scientific information that's available at this point in time, it isn't advisable to use creatine without the approval of a physician.

Q: Will caffeine improve my workouts?

A: Caffeine – a stimulant of the central nervous system – is perhaps the most widely used drug in the world. It's a component of tea, coffee, chocolate and soft drinks as well as pills to lose weight and combat drowsiness. It has no significant nutritional value.

Interest in the use of caffeine as a performance enhancer – or "ergogenic aid" – was primarily inspired by two studies that were published in the late 1970s. In those studies, caffeine produced significant improvements in endurance (in cycling). To date, numerous studies done in a laboratory setting have shown that caffeine increases performance in cycling and running for durations of roughly 5 - 20 minutes. But studies done outside a laboratory have found mixed results. When consumed in low doses, caffeine can improve perception, increase alertness, decrease reaction time and reduce anxiety levels.

In low doses, caffeine doesn't pose any serious risks for healthy individuals; when consumed in high doses, caffeine has the potential for many adverse side effects such as anxiety, jitters, tremors, inability to focus, gastrointestinal distress, diarrhea, insomnia, irritability and "withdrawal headache." Since caffeine is a potent diuretic (which increases the production of urine), there has been some concern that it can increase the risk of dehydration – a major fear during physical activity, especially in a hot, humid environment. Individuals who have pre-existing ulcer conditions or are prone to stomach distress should avoid caffeine.

Q: Should I take ephedrine before I do physical activities?

A: Ephedrine – also known as "ephedra" – is an over-the-counter herbal stimulant that's found in many cold and flu medications as well as supplements that are marketed for weight loss. Understand that ephedrine is an amphetamine-like compound that has many adverse side effects including dizziness and headaches. Ephedrine also increases your heart rate and blood pressure. Needless to say, it isn't in your best interests to elevate your heart rate and blood pressure and then do some type of physical exertion. In one study, researchers concluded that ephedrine produces a significant increase in blood pressure and when taken prior to intense physical activity, exposes individuals to "cardiovascular risks." Of greater concern is the combination of ephedrine and caffeine. One study found that when these two stimulants were ingested together, subjects increased their resting systolic blood pressure (the upper number) by an average of 18 milliliters of mercury – from 138 to 156.

The use of ephedrine also increases the potential for dehydration and has been linked to seizures, strokes and heart attacks. Since 1994, the Food and Drug Administration has received *more than 800 reports* of adverse side effects from ephedrine including *at least 160 deaths* (29 of which occurred in 2003).

Because of these and other risks, the sale of dietary supplements that contain ephedra was banned in the United States on April 12, 2004. The ban doesn't include over-the-counter or prescription drugs.

Q: Is it safe to use herbs and other nutritional supplements that are natural?

A: First of all, remember that the Food and Drug Administration doesn't regulate herbs and other nutritional supplements for safety, effectiveness, purity or potency. Due to this lack of federal oversight, you really don't know exactly what's in the products. In one study, researchers analyzed 75 different nutritional products and found that seven (9.33%) contained substances that weren't shown on the labels. Moreover, the active ingredient may be higher or lower than the amount listed on the label. Herbs and other nutritional supplements may also contain contaminants – most likely from the manufacturing process – such as aluminum, lead, mercury and tin.

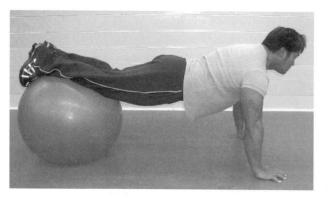

Photo 20-6: Exercising on stability balls can be used to provide variety to workouts.

Many herbs and other nutritional supplements are promoted as "natural." Because a product claims to be "natural" or have "natural" ingredients doesn't mean that it's necessarily safe. Dirt is "natural" but that doesn't mean it's safe to eat. The truth is that many "natural" substances can be quite harmful including high-potency doses of some vitamins, minerals and certain herbs. For instance, large doses of the natural stimulants found in ginseng can cause hypertension, insomnia, depression and skin blemishes. There are similar safety concerns with high-potency enzymes, inert glandulars and animal extracts. One final point is that it's difficult to predict how some herbs interact with prescription and over-the-counter medications (as well as other nutritional supplements).

Finally, remember that many herbs and other nutritional supplements come with express or implied disease-related claims and are marketed for specific therapeutic purposes for which there may not be valid scientific proof. In one study, researchers reviewed all of the clinical trials that were published in 1966 - 1992 and compared the pertinent human and/or animal studies to that of the manufacturer's claims. It was found that 8 of the 19 products (42%) had no published scientific evidence to support the promotional claims. Another 6 of the 19 (32%) were judged as being marketed in a misleading manner. The fact of the matter is that the majority of herbs and other nutritional supplements have no recognized role in nutrition.

APPENDIX A: BASIC ANATOMY – FRONT VIEW

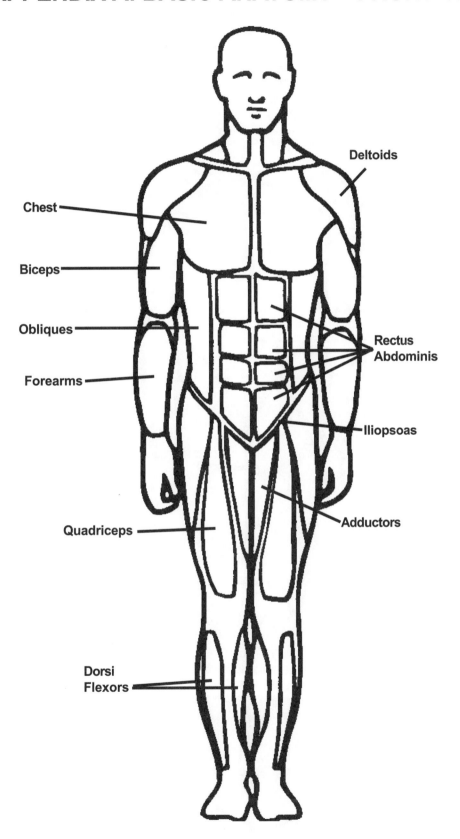

Chest

Biceps

Obliques

Forearms

Quadriceps

Dorsi
Flexors

Deltoids

Rectus
Abdominis

Iliopsoas

Adductors

Artwork courtesy of Cybex International, Inc.

APPENDIX B: BASIC ANATOMY – BACK VIEW

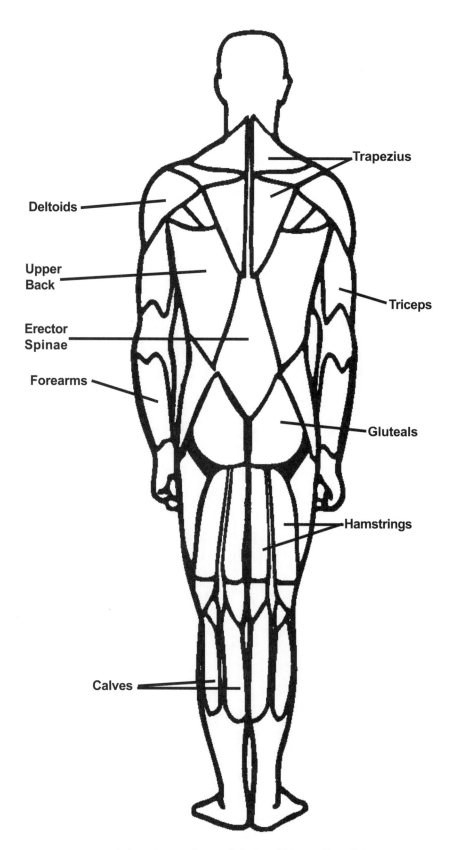

Trapezius

Deltoids

Upper
Back

Triceps

Erector
Spinae

Forearms

Gluteals

Hamstrings

Calves

Artwork courtesy of Cybex International, Inc.

APPENDIX C: SAMPLE WORKOUT CARD
FOR AEROBIC TRAINING

NAME:

DATE	BODY WEIGHT	ACTIVITY	TIME	DISTANCE	PACE	EXERCISE HEART RATE	RECOVERY HEART RATE

AGE-PREDICTED MAXIMUM HEART RATE:	HEART-RATE TRAINING ZONE: -

APPENDIX D: SAMPLE WORKOUT CARD
FOR SINGLE-SET TRAINING

NAME:		DATE													
		BW													
	EXERCISE	REPS	wt/reps	wt/reps	wt/reps	wt/reps	wt/reps	wt/reps	wt/reps	wt/reps	wt/reps	wt/reps	wt/reps	wt/reps
Hips (1)															
Upper Legs (2)															
Lower Legs (1)															
Chest (2)															
Upper Back (2)															
Shoulders (2)															
Upper Arm (2)															
Lower Arm (2)															
Abdominals (1)															
Lower Back (1)															
Other															

APPENDIX E: SAMPLE WORKOUT CARD
FOR MULTIPLE-SET TRAINING

NAME:		DATE												
		BW												
	EXERCISE	REPS	wt reps	wt reps	wt reps	wt reps	wt reps	wt reps	wt reps	wt reps	wt reps	wt reps	wt reps	wt reps
Hips (1)														
Upper Legs (2)														
Lower Legs (1)														
Chest (2)														
Upper Back (2)														
Shoulders (2)														
Upper Arm (2)														
Lower Arm (2)														
Abdominals (1)														
Lower Back (1)														
Other														

BIBLIOGRAPHY

Allison, DB, and SB Heymsfield. 1998. "Natural" therapeutics for weight loss: garden of slender delights or dangerous alchemy? *Nutrition & the M. D.* 24 (1): 1-3.

American College of Sports Medicine [ACSM]. 2000. *ACSM's guidelines for graded exercise testing and exercise prescription. 6th ed*. Philadelphia, PA: Lippincott Williams & Wilkins.

American Council on Exercise [ACE]. 1991. *Personal trainer manual: the resource for fitness instructors*. San Diego, CA: ACE.

Anderson, O. 2002. You do have a "fat-burning zone," but do you really want to go there to "burn off" fat? *Running Research News* 18 (2): 7-10.

Andrews, JG, JG Hay and CL Vaughan. 1983. Knee shear forces during a squat exercise using a barbell and a weight machine. In *Biomechanics VIII-B*, ed. H Matsui and K Kobayashi, 923-927. Champaign, IL: Human Kinetics Publishers, Inc.

Arendt, EA. 1984. Strength development: a comparison of resistive exercise techniques. *Contemporary Orthopaedics* 9 (3): 67-72.

Asimov, I. 1992. *The human body: its structure and operation. Revised ed*. New York, NY: Mentor.

Asmussen, E. 1952. Positive and negative muscular work. *Acta Physiologica Scandinavica* 28: 364-382.

Astrand, I. 1960. Aerobic work capacity in men and women with special reference to age. *Acta Physiologica Scandinavica* 49 (Supplementum 169): 1-92.

Astrand, P-O, and K Rodahl. 1977. *Textbook of work physiology. 2d ed*. New York, NY: McGraw-Hill Book Company.

Barron, RL, and GJ Vanscoy. 1993. Natural products and the athlete: facts and folklore. *Annals of Pharmacotherapy* 27 (5): 607-615.

Bates, B, M Wolf and J Blunk. 1990. *Vanderbilt University strength and conditioning manual*. Nashville, TN: Vanderbilt University.

Behm, DG, K Anderson and RS Curnew. 2002. Muscle force and activation under stable and unstable conditions. *Journal of Strength and Conditioning Research* 16 (3): 416-422.

Ben-Ezra, V. 1992. Assessing physical fitness. In *The Stairmaster fitness handbook*, ed. JA Peterson and CX Bryant, 91-108. Indianapolis, IN: Masters Press.

Berlin, I, D Warot, G Aymard, E Acquaviva, M Legrand, B Labarthe, I Peyron, B Diquet and P Lechat. 2001. Pharmacodynamics and pharmacokinetics of single nasal (5 mg and 10 mg) and oral (50 mg) doses of ephedrine in healthy subjects. *European Journal of Clinical Pharmacology* 57 (6-7): 447-455.

Bishop, D. 2003. Warm up I: potential mechanisms and the effects of passive warm up on exercise performance. *Sports Medicine* 33 (6): 439-454.

_____. 2003. Warm up II: performance changes following active warm up and how to structure the warm up. *Sports Medicine* 33 (7): 483-498.

Bolotte, CP. 1998. Creatine supplementation in athletes: benefits and potential risks. *Journal of the Louisiana State Medical Society* 150 (July): 325-328.

Bouchard, C. 1983. Genetics of physiological fitness and motor performance. *Exercise and Sport Sciences Reviews* 11: 306-339.

Boyer, BT. 1990. A comparison of the effects of three strength training programs on women. *Journal of Applied Sport Science Research* 4 (3): 88-94.

Braith, RW, JE Graves, ML Pollock, SH Leggett, DM Carpenter and AB Colvin. 1989. Comparison of 2 vs 3 days/week of variable resistance training during 10- and 18-week programs. *International Journal of Sports Medicine* 10 (6): 450-454.

Brand-Miller, J, S Colagiuri, TMS Wolever and K Foster-Powell. 1999. *The glucose revolution*. New York, NY: Marlowe & Company.

Bryant, CX, BA Franklin and JM Conviser. 2002. *Exercise testing and program design: a fitness professional's handbook*. Monterey, CA: Exercise Science Publishers.

Bryant, CX, and JA Peterson. 1992. Estimating aerobic fitness. *Fitness Management* 9 (August): 36-39.

Bryant, CX, and JA Peterson. 1994. Strength training for the heart? *Fitness Management* 10 (February): 32-34.

Bryant, CX, JA Peterson and RJ Hagen. 1994. Weight loss: unfolding the truth. *Fitness Management* 10 (May): 42-44.

Bryant, CX, and JA Peterson. 1996. All exercise is not equal. *Fitness Management* 12 (July): 32-34.

Brzycki, MM. 1995. *A practical approach to strength training. 3d ed*. New York, NY: McGraw-Hill/Contemporary.

_____. 1997. *Cross training for fitness*. New York, NY: McGraw-Hill/Contemporary.

_____. 1998. Quality REPS. *Fitness Management* 14 (June): 44-46.

_____. 1999. Free weights and machines. *Fitness Management* 15 (June): 36-37, 40.

_____. 2000. Creatine supplementation: effective and safe? *Master Trainer* 10: 11-18.

_____. 2002. Spicing up strength-training programs with variety. *Fitness Management* 18 (June): 40, 42, 44.

_____. 2004. 10 myths about strength training. *Fitness Management* (YMCA) 19 (January): 43-48.

_____. 2004. 10 myths about cardio training. *Fitness Management* (YMCA) 20 (June): 28-31.

_____. 2004. 10 myths about flexibility training. *Fitness Management* (YMCA) 20 (August): 38-41.

Bubb, WJ. 1992. Nutrition. In *Health fitness instructor's handbook, 2d ed*, by ET Howley and BD Franks, 95-114. Champaign, IL: Human Kinetics Publishers, Inc.

_____. 1992. Relative leanness. In *Health fitness instructor's handbook, 2d ed*, by ET Howley and BD Franks, 115-130. Champaign, IL: Human Kinetics Publishers, Inc.

Burke, LM, GR Collier and M Hargreaves. 1993. Muscle glycogen storage after prolonged exercise: effect of the glycemic index of carbohydrate feeding. *Journal of Applied Physiology* 75 (2): 1019-1023.

Butterfield, G. 1991. Amino acids and high protein diets. In *Perspectives in exercise science and sports medicine, volume 4*, ed. DR Lamb and M Williams, 87-122. Indianapolis, IN: Brown & Benchmark.

Calder, AW, PD Chilibeck, CE Webber and DG Sale. 1994. Comparison of whole and split weight training routines in young women. *Canadian Journal of Applied Physiology* 19 (2): 185-199.

Cappozzo, A, F Felici, F Figura and F Gazzani. 1985. Lumbar spine loading during half-squat exercises. *Medicine and Science in Sports and Exercise* 17 (5): 613-620.

Carpinelli, RN. 1999. Serious strength training. *High Intensity Training Newsletter* 9 (6): 9-10.

_____. 2001. The science of strength training. *Master Trainer* 11 (4): 10-17.

Carpinelli, RN, and RM Otto. 1998. Strength training. Single versus multiple sets. *Sports Medicine* 26 (2): 73-84.

Carpinelli, RN, RM Otto and RA Winett. 2004. A critical analysis of the ACSM position stand on resistance training: insufficient evidence to support recommended training protocols. *Journal of Exercise Physiologyonline* 7 (3): 1-60.

Carter, JEL, and BH Heath. 1971. Somatotype methodology and kinesiology research. *Kinesiology Review* 1: 10-19.

Chestnut, JL, and D Docherty. 1999. The effects of 4 and 10 repetition maximum weight-training protocols on neuromuscular adaptations in untrained men. *Journal of Strength and Conditioning Research* 13 (4): 353-359.

Cheuvront, SN. 1999. The Zone Diet and athletic performance. *Sports Medicine* 27 (4): 213-228.

City of New York Department of Consumer Affairs. 1992. *Magic muscle pills!! Health and fitness quackery in nutrition supplements.* New York, NY: Department of Consumer Affairs.

Clark, N. 1990. *Nancy Clark's sports nutrition guidebook.* Champaign, IL: Leisure Press.

Clarkson, PM, and ES Rawson. 1999. Nutritional supplements to increase muscle mass. *Clinical Reviews in Food Science and Nutrition* 39 (4): 317-328.

Clausen, JP. 1977. Effect of physical training on cardiovascular adjustments to exercise in man. *Physiological Reviews* 57 (4): 779-815.

Coleman, E. 2001. Being supplement savvy. *Sports Medicine Digest* 24 (4): 46-47.

Colliander, EB, and PA Tesch. 1990. Effects of eccentric and concentric muscle actions in resistance training. *Acta Physiologica Scandinavica* 140 (1): 31-39.

Costill, DL, GP Dalsky and WJ Fink. 1978. Effects of caffeine ingestion on metabolism and exercise performance. *Medicine and Science in Sports and Exercise* 10 (3): 155-158.

Crouch, JE. 1978. *Functional human anatomy. 3d ed.* Philadelphia, PA: Lea & Febiger.

Cummings, S, ES Parham and GW Strain. 2002. Position of the American Dietetic Association: weight management. *Journal of the American Dietetic Association* 102 (8): 1145-1155.

DeLateur, BJ, JF Lehman and R Giaconi. 1976. Mechanical work and fatigue: their roles in the development of muscle work capacity. *Archives of Physical Medicine and Rehabilitation* 57 (1): 319-324.

DeLorme, TL. 1945. Restoration of muscle power by heavy resistance exercise. *Journal of Bone and Joint Surgery* 27 (October): 645-667.

DeLorme, TL, and AL Watkins. 1948. Techniques of progressive resistance exercise. *Archives of Physical Medicine* 27 (October): 645-667.

deVries, HA. 1974. *Physiology of exercise for physical education and athletics. 2d ed.* Dubuque, IA: William C. Brown.

Dons, B, K Bollerup, F Bonde-Petersen and S Hancke. 1979. The effect of weight-lifting exercise related to muscle fiber composition and muscle cross-sectional area in humans. *European Journal of Applied Physiology* 40 (2): 95-106.

Dudley, GA, PA Tesch, BJ Miller and P Buchanan. 1991. Importance of eccentric actions in performance adaptations to resistance training. *Aviation, Space, and Environmental Medicine* 62 (6): 543-550.

Durak, E. 1987. Physical performance responses to muscle lengthening and weight training exercises in young women. *Journal of Applied Sport Science Research* 1 (3): 60.

Enoka, RM. 1994. *Neuromechanical basis of kinesiology. 2d ed*. Champaign, IL: Human Kinetics Publishers, Inc.

_____. 1988. Muscle strength and its development. *Sports Medicine* 6 (3): 146-168.

Ernst, E. 1998. Harmless herbs? A review of the recent literature. *The American Journal of Medicine* 104 (February): 170-178.

Esbjornsson, M, C Sylven, I Holm and E Jansson. 1993. Fast twitch fibres may predict anaerobic performance in both females and males. *International Journal of Sports Medicine* 14 (5): 257-263.

Falk, B, R Burstein, I Ashkanazi, O Spilberg, J Alter, E Zylber-Katz, A Rubenstein, N Bashan and Y Shapiro. 1989. The effects of caffeine ingestion on physical performance after prolonged exercise. *European Journal of Applied Physiology* 59 (3): 168-173.

Falk, B, R Burstein, J Rosenblum, Y Shapiro, E Zylber-Katz and N Bashan. 1990. Effects of caffeine ingestion on body fluid balance and thermoregulation during exercise. *Canadian Journal of Physiology and Pharmacology* 68 (7): 889-892.

Farley, D. 1993. Dietary supplements: making sure hype doesn't overwhelm science. *FDA Consumer* 27 (November): 8-13.

Feigenbaum, MS, and ML Pollock. 1997. Strength training: rationale for current guidelines for adult fitness programs. *The Physician and Sportsmedicine* 25 (2): 44-46, 49, 54-56, 63-64.

_____. 1999. Prescription of resistance training for health and disease. *Medicine and Science in Sports and Exercise* 31 (1): 38-45.

Fellingham, GW, ES Roundy, AG Fisher and GR Bryce. 1978. Caloric cost of walking and running. *Medicine and Science in Sports and Exercise* 10 (2): 132-136.

Fincher II, G. 2000. Less is more in resistance training. *Biomechanics* 7 (11): 43-44, 46, 48, 50, 52.

Fink, KJ, and B Worthington-Roberts. 1995. Nutritional considerations for exercise. In *The Stairmaster fitness handbook, 2d ed*, ed. JA Peterson and CX Bryant, 205-228. St. Louis, MO: Wellness Bookshelf.

Fox, EL, and DK Mathews. 1981. *The physiological basis of physical education and athletics. 3d ed*. Philadelphia, PA: Saunders College Publishing.

Fox, EL. 1984. Physiology of exercise and physical fitness. In *Sports medicine*, ed. R. H. Strauss, 381-456. Philadelphia: W. B. Saunders Company.

Frankel, VH, and M Nordin. 1980. *Basic biomechanics of the skeletal system*. Philadelphia, PA: Lea & Febiger.

Fukunaga, T, M Miyatani, M Tachi, M Kouzaki, Y Kawakami and H Kanehisa. 2001. Muscle volume is a major determinant of joint torque in humans. *Acta Physiologica Scandinavica* 172 (4): 249-255.

Garrett Jr, WE, and TR Malone, eds. 1988. *Muscle development: nutritional alternatives to anabolic steroids*. Columbus, OH: Ross Laboratories.

Goldberg, AL, JD Etlinger, DF Goldspink and C Jablecki. 1975. Mechanism of work-induced hypertrophy of skeletal muscle. *Medicine and Science in Sports* 7 (3): 248-261.

Graham, AS, and RC Hatton. 1999. Creatine: a review of efficacy and safety. *Journal of the American Pharmaceutical Association* 39 (6): 803-810.

Graham, TE. 2001. Caffeine, coffee and ephedrine: impact on exercise performance and metabolism. *Canadian Journal of Applied Physiology* 26 (supplement): S103-S119.

Graham, TE, and LL Spriet. 1996. Caffeine and exercise performance. *Sports Science Exchange* 9 (1): 1-5.

Graves, JE, and ML Pollock. 1995. Understanding the physiological basis of muscular fitness. In *The Stairmaster fitness handbook, 2d ed*, ed. JA Peterson and CX Bryant, 67-80. St. Louis, MO: Wellness Bookshelf.

Graves, JE, ML Pollock, SH Leggett, RW Braith, DM Carpenter and LE Bishop. 1988. Effect of reduced training frequency on muscular strength. *International Journal of Sports Medicine* 9 (5): 316-319.

Graves, JE, ML Pollock, AE Jones, AB Colvin and SH Leggett. 1989. Specificity of limited range of motion variable resistance training. *Medicine and Science in Sports and Exercise* 21 (1): 84-89.

Graves, JE, ML Pollock, D Foster, SH Leggett, DM Carpenter, R Vuoso and A Jones. 1990. Effect of training frequency and specificity on isometric lumbar extension strength. *Spine* 15 (6): 504-509.

Guthrie, HA. 1983. *Introductory nutrition. 5th ed*. St. Louis, MO: The C. V. Mosby Company.

Hakkinen, K, A Pakarinen and M Kallinen. 1992. Neuromuscular adaptations and serum hormones in women during short-term intensive strength training. *European Journal of Applied Physiology* 64 (2): 106-111.

van Handel, P. 1983. Caffeine. In *Ergogenic aids in sport*, ed ML Williams, 128-163. Champaign, IL: Human Kinetics Publishers.

Hass, CJ, L Garzarella, D De Hoyos and ML Pollock. 2000. Single versus multiple sets in long-term recreational weightlifters. *Medicine and Science in Sports and Exercise* 32 (1): 235-242.

Hather, BM, PA Tesch, P Buchanan and GA Dudley. 1991. Influence of eccentric actions on skeletal muscle adaptations to resistance training. *Acta Physiologica Scandinavica* 143 (2): 177-185.

Hay, JG, and JG Reid. 1988. *Anatomy, mechanics, and human motion. 2d ed.* Englewood Cliffs, NJ: Prentice-Hall, Inc.

Hay, JG, JG Andrews and CL Vaughn. 1983. Effects of lifting rate on elbow torques exerted during arm curl exercises. *Medicine and Science in Sports and Exercise* 15 (1): 63-71.

Hellebrandt, FA. 1958. Special review: application of the overload principle to muscle training in man. *American Journal of Physical Medicine* 37 (5): 278-283.

Hellebrandt, FA, and SJ Houtz. 1956. Mechanisms of muscle training in man: experimental demonstration of the overload principle. *Physical Therapy Review* 36 (6): 371-383.

Hempel, LS, and CL Wells. 1985. Cardiorespiratory cost of the Nautilus express circuit. *The Physician and Sportsmedicine* 13 (4): 86-86, 91-97.

Herbert, RD, and M Gabriel. 2002. Effects of stretching before and after exercising on muscle soreness and risk of injury: systematic review. *British Medical Journal* 325: 468-472.

Herbert, V, and GJ Subak-Sharpe, eds. 1990. *The Mount Sinai School of Medicine complete book of nutrition.* New York, NY: St. Martin's Press.

Hickson, RC, C Kanakis, JR Davis, AM Moore and S Rich. 1982. Reduced training duration effects on aerobic power, endurance and cardiac growth. *Journal of Applied Physiology* 53 (1): 225-229.

Higbie, EJ, KJ Cureton, GL Warren III and BM Prior. 1996. Effects of concentric and eccentric training on muscle strength, cross-sectional area, and neural activation. *Journal of Applied Physiology* 81 (5): 2173-2181.

High, DM, ET Howley and BD Franks. 1989. The effects of static stretching and warm-up on prevention of delayed-onset muscle soreness. *Research Quarterly for Exercise and Sport* 60 (4): 357-361.

Hill, AV. 1922. The maximum work and mechanical efficiency in human muscles, and their most economical speed. *Journal of Physiology* 56: 19-41.

Hirt, S. 1967. Historical bases for therapeutic exercise. *American Journal of Physical Medicine* 46 (1): 32-38.

Hoeger, WWK. 1988. *Principles and labs for physical fitness and wellness.* Englewood, CO: Morton Publishing Co.

Hoffman, B. 1939. *Weight lifting.* York, PA: Strength & Health Publishing Co.

Houston, ME. 1999. Gaining weight: the scientific basis of increasing skeletal muscle mass. *Canadian Journal of Applied Physiology* 24 (4): 305-316.

Howley, ET, and BD Franks. 1992. *Health fitness instructor's handbook. 2d ed.* Champaign, IL: Human Kinetics Publishers, Inc.

Howley, ET, and M Glover. 1974. The caloric costs of running and walking one mile for men and women. *Medicine and Science in Sports and Exercise* 6 (4): 235-237.

Hurley, BF, DR Seals, AA Ehsani, L-J Cartier, GP Dalsky, JM Hagberg and JO Holloszy. 1984. Effects of high-intensity strength training on cardiovascular function. *Medicine and Science in Sports and Exercise* 16 (5): 483-488.

Hurley, D. 2004. As ephedra ban nears, a race to sell the last supplies. *The New York Times* (April 11): 23.

Huxley, HE. 1958. The contraction of muscle. *Scientific American* 199 (5): 66-82.

Ikai, M, and T Fukunaga. 1965. The mechanism of muscular contraction. *Scientific American* 213 (6): 18-27.

Ivy, JL. 1991. Muscle glycogen synthesis before and after exercise. *Sports Medicine* 11 (1): 6-19.

_____. 2001. Dietary strategies to promote glycogen synthesis after exercise. *Canadian Journal of Applied Physiology* 26 (supplement): S236-S245.

Ivy, JL, DL Costill, WJ Fink and RW Lower. 1979. Influence of caffeine and carbohydrate feedings on endurance performance. *Medicine and Science in Sports and Exercise* 11 (1): 6-11.

Jacobs, I, H Pasternak and DG Bell. 2003. Effects of ephedrine, caffeine, and their combination on muscular endurance. *Medicine and Science in Sports and Exercise* 35 (6): 987-994.

Jakicic, JM, K Clark, E Coleman, JE Donnelly, J Foreyt, E Melanson, J Volek and SL Volpe. 2001. ACSM position stand on the appropriate intervention strategies for weight loss and prevention of weight regain for adults. *Medicine and Science in Sports and Exercise* 33 (12): 2145-2156.

Jones, A. 1970. *Nautilus training principles, bulletin #1.* DeLand, FL: Arthur Jones Productions.

_____. 1971. *Nautilus training principles, bulletin #2.* DeLand, FL: Arthur Jones Productions.

_____. 1993. *The lumbar spine, the cervical spine and the knee: testing and rehabilitation.* Ocala, FL: MedX Corporation.

Jones, A, ML Pollock, JE Graves, M Fulton, W Jones, M MacMillan, DD Baldwin and J Cirulli. 1988. *Safe, spe-*

cific testing and rehabilitative exercise of the muscles of the lumbar spine. Santa Barbara, CA: Sequoia Communications.

Jones, NL, N McCartney and AJ McComas, eds. 1986. *Human muscle power.* Champaign, IL: Human Kinetics Publishers, Inc.

Juhn, MS, JW O'Kane and DM Vinci. 1999. Oral creatine supplementation in male collegiate athletes: a survey of dosing habits and side effects. *Journal of the American Dietetic Association* 99 (5): 593-595.

Juhn, MS, and M Tarnopolsky. 1998. Potential side effects of oral creatine supplementation: a critical review. *Clinical Journal of Sports Medicine* 8 (4): 298-304.

Kamber, M, N Baume, M Savgy and L River. 2001. Nutritional supplements as a source for positive doping cases? *International Journal of Sport Nutrition and Exercise Metabolism* 11 (2): 258-263.

Kaneko, M, PV Komi and O Aura. 1984. Mechanical efficiency of concentric and eccentric exercises performed with medium to fast contraction rates. *Scandinavian Journal of Sport Science* 6: 15-20.

Karlsson, J, PV Komi and JHT Viitasalo. 1979. Muscle strength and muscle characteristics in monozygous and dizygous twins. *Acta Physiologica Scandinavica* 106 (3): 319-325.

Katch, FI, PM Clarkson, WA Kroll and T McBride. 1984. Effects of sit up exercise training on adipose cell size and adiposity. *Research Quarterly for Exercise and Sport* 55 (3): 242-247

Katzmarzyk, PT, RM Malina, L Perusse, T Rice, MA Province, DC Rao and C Bouchard. 2000. Familial resemblance for physique: heritabilities for somatotype components. *Annals of Human Biology* 27 (5): 467-477.

Kaczkowski, W, DL Montgomery, AW Taylor and V Klissouras. 1982. The relationship between muscle fiber composition and maximal anaerobic power and capacity. *Journal of Sports Medicine* 22 (4): 407-413.

Klein, KK. 1962. Squats right. *Scholastic Coach* 32 (2): 36-38, 70-71.

Klissouras, V. 1971. Heritability of adaptive variation. *Journal of Applied Physiology* 31 (3): 338-344.

_____. 1973. Genetic aspects of physical fitness. *Journal of Sports Medicine* 13: 164-170.

_____. 1997. Heritability of adaptive variation: an old problem revisited. *The Journal of Sports Medicine and Physical Fitness* 37 (1): 1-6.

Koshy, KM, E Griswold and EE Schneeberger. 1999. Interstitial nephritis in patient taking creatine. *New England Journal of Medicine* 340 (10): 814-815.

Kraemer, WJ. 1992. Involvement of eccentric muscle action may optimize adaptations to resistance training. *Sports Science Exchange* 4 (6): 1-4.

Kreahling, L. 2004. New thoughts about when not to stretch. *The New York Times* (April 27): F5.

Krieder, RB, V Miriel and E Bertun. 1993. Amino acid supplementation and exercise performance: analysis of the proposed ergogenic value. *Sports Medicine* 16 (3): 190-209.

Kris-Etherton, PM. 1989. The facts and fallacies of nutritional supplements for athletes. *Sports Science Exchange* 2 (8): 1-4.

Kuehl, K, L Goldberg and D Elliot. 1998. Renal insufficiency after creatine supplementation in a college football athlete. *Medicine and Science in Sports and Exercise* 30 (5): S235.

Lamb, DR. 1984. *Physiology of exercise: responses & adaptations. 2d ed.* New York, NY: MacMillan Publishing Company.

Lambrinides, T. 1990. High intensity training and overtraining. *High Intensity Training Newsletter* 2 (2): 9-10.

Leistner, KE. 1986. The quality repetition. *The Steel Tip* 2 (June): 6-7.

Lieber, DC, RL Lieber and WC Adams. 1989. Effects of run-training and swim-training at similar absolute intensities on treadmill VO$_2$ max. *Medicine and Science in Sports and Exercise* 21 (6): 655-661.

Lillegard, WA, and JD Terrio. 1994. Appropriate strength training. *Sports Medicine* 78 (2): 457-477.

Lomangino, K. 2002. More doubt cast on value of pre-exercise stretching. *Sports Medicine Digest* 24 (10): 109, 111-112.

Londeree, BR, and ML Moeschberger. 1982. Effect of age and other factors on maximal heart rate. *Research Quarterly for Exercise and Sport* 53 (4): 297-304.

Lowenthal, DT, and Y Karni. 1990. The nutritional needs of athletes. In *The Mount Sinai School of Medicine complete book of nutrition*, ed. V Herbert and GJ Subak-Sharpe, 396-414. New York, NY: St. Martin's Press.

Lukaski, HC. 1995. Micronutrients (magnesium, zinc, and copper): are mineral supplements needed for athletes? *International Journal of Sports Nutrition* 5 (supplement): S74-S83.

MacDougall, D, and DG Sale. 1981. Continuous vs. interval training: a review for the athlete and coach. *Canadian Journal of Applied Sport Sciences* 6 (2): 87-92.

Mannie, K. 2001. *Michigan State summer manual.* East Lansing, MI: Michigan State University.

_____. 1988. Key factors in program organization. *High Intensity Training Newsletter* 1 (1): 4-5.

Manore, MM, SI Barr and GE Butterfield. 2000. Joint position statement by the American College of Sports Medicine, American Dietetic Association and Dieticians of Canada on nutrition and athletic performance. *Medicine and Science in Sports and Exercise* 32 (12): 2130-2145.

McArdle, WD, FI Katch and VL Katch. 1986. *Exercise physiology: energy, nutrition and human performance. 2d ed.* Philadelphia, PA: Lea & Febiger.

McArdle, WD, JR Margel, DJ Delio, M Toner and JM Chase. 1978. Specificity of run training on VO_2 max and heart rate changes during running and swimming. *Medicine and Science in Sports and Exercise* 10 (1): 16-20.

McCarthy, JP, JC Agre, BK Graf, MA Pozniak and AC Vailas. 1995. Compatibility of adaptive responses with combining strength and endurance training. *Medicine and Science in Sports and Exercise* 27 (3): 429-436.

McCarthy, P. 1989. How much protein do athletes really need? *The Physician and Sportsmedicine* 17 (5): 170-175.

Mentzer, M. 1993. *Heavy duty.* Venice, CA: Mike Mentzer.

Messier, SP, and M Dill. 1985. Alterations in strength and maximal oxygen uptake consequent to Nautilus circuit weight training. *Research Quarterly for Exercise and Sport* 56 (4): 345-351.

Moritani, T, and HA deVries. 1979. Neural factors vs hypertrophy in the course of muscle strength gain. *American Journal of Physical Medicine and Rehabilitation* 58 (3): 115-130.

Mujika, I, and S Padilla. 1997. Creatine supplementation as an ergogenic aid for sports performance in highly trained athletes: a critical review. *International Journal of Sports Medicine* 18 (7): 491-496.

National Collegiate Athletic Association [NCAA]. 1991. No miracles found in many "natural potions." *NCAA News* 28 (July 17): 7.

NCAA Committee on Competitive Safeguards and Medical Aspects of Sports. 1992. Ergogenic aids and nutrition. Overland Park, KS: NCAA memorandum (August 6).

National Research Council, Committee on Diet and Health, Food and Nutrition Board. 1989. *Diet and health: implications for reducing chronic disease risk.* Washington, DC: National Academy Press.

Parascrampuria, J, K Schwartz and R Petesch. 1998. Quality control of dehydroepiandrosterone dietary supplements. *Journal of the American Medical Association* 280 (8): 1565.

Paton, CD, WG Hopkins and L Vollebregt. 2001. Little effect of caffeine ingestion on repeated sprints in team-sport athletes. *Medicine and Science in Sports and Exercise* 33 (5): 822-825.

Pecci, MA, and JA Lombardo. 2000. Performance-enhancing supplements. *Physical Medicine and Rehabilitation Clinics of North America* 11 (4): 949-960.

Peterson, JA, ed. 1978. *Total fitness: the Nautilus way.* West Point, NY: Leisure Press.

Peterson, JA, and CX Bryant, eds. 1992. *The Stairmaster fitness handbook.* Indianapolis, IN: Masters Press.

Peterson, JA, and CX Bryant, eds. 1995. *The Stairmaster fitness handbook. 2d ed.* St. Louis, MO: Wellness Bookshelf.

Peterson, JA, and WL Westcott. 1990. Stronger by the minute. *Fitness Management* 6 (June): 22-24.

Philen, RM, DI Ortiz, SB Auerbach and H Falk. 1992. Survey of advertising for nutritional supplements in health and bodybuilding magazines. *Journal of the American Medical Association* 268 (8): 1008-1011.

Piehl, K. 1974. Glycogen storage and depletion in human skeletal muscle fibers. *Acta Physiologica Scandinavica* (Supplementum 402): 1-32.

Pipes, TV. 1989. *The steroid alternative.* Placerville, CA: Sierra Gold Graphics.

———. 1979. High intensity, not high speed. *Athletic Journal* 59 (December): 60, 62.

———. 1988. A.C.T. - The steroid alternative. *Scholastic Coach* 57 (January): 106, 108-109, 112.

Pitts, EH. 1992. Pills, powders, potions and persuasions. *Fitness Management* 9 (November): 34-35.

Pollock, ML. 1973. The quantification of endurance training programs. In *Exercise and sport sciences reviews*, ed. JH Wilmore, 155-188. New York, NY: Academic Press.

Pollock, ML, JE Graves, DM Carpenter, D Foster, SH Leggett and MN Fulton. 1993. The lumbar musculature: testing and conditioning for rehabilitation. In *Rehabilitation of the spine*, eds. SH Hochchuler, RD Guyer and HB Cotler, 263-284. St. Louis: Mosby, Inc.

Pollock, ML, J Dimmick, HS Miller, Z Kendrick and AC Linnerud. 1975. Effects of mode of training on cardiovascular function and body composition of middle-aged men. *Medicine and Science in Sports and Exercise* 7 (2): 139-145.

Pollock, ML, GA Gaesser, JD Butcher, J-P Despres, RK Dishman, BA Franklin and CE Garber. 1998. ACSM position stand on the recommended quantity and quality of exercise for developing and maintaining cardiorespiratory and muscular fitness, and flexibility in healthy adults. *Medicine and Science in Sports and Exercise* 30 (6): 975-991.

Porcari, JP. 1994. Fat-burning exercise: fit or farce. *Fitness Management* 10 (July): 40-41.

Porcari, J, and J Curtis. 1996. Can you work strength and aerobics at the same time? *Fitness Management* 12 (June): 26-29.

Pritchard, NR, and PA Kalra. 1998. Renal dysfunction accompanying oral creatine supplements. *Lancet* 351: 1252-1253.

Rasch, PJ. 1989. *Kinesiology and applied anatomy. 7th ed.* Philadelphia, PA: Lea & Febiger.

Rasmussen, BB, KD Tipton, SL Miller, SE Wolf and RR Wolfe. 2000. An oral essential amino acid-carbohydrate supplement enhances muscle protein anabolism after resistance exercise. *Journal of Applied Physiology* 88: 386-392.

Reid, CM, RA Yeater and IH Ullrich. 1987. Weight training and strength, cardiorespiratory functioning and body composition in men. *British Journal of Sports Medicine* 21 (1): 40-44.

Riley, DP. 1982. *Strength training by the experts. 2d ed.* West Point, NY: Leisure Press.

_____. 1979. Speed of exercise versus speed of movement. *Scholastic Coach* 48 (May/June): 90, 92-93, 97-98.

_____. 1980. Time and intensity: keys to maximum strength gains. *Scholastic Coach* 50 (November): 65-66, 74-75.

_____. 1982. Guidelines for strength program. *Scholastic Coach* 51 (May/June): 64-65, 80.

Riley, DP, and R Wright. 2004. *Houston Texans strength & conditioning program.* Houston, TX: Houston Texans.

Roberts, DF. 1984. Genetic determinants of sports performance. In *Sport and human genetics*, ed. RM Malina and C Bouchard, 105-121. Champaign, IL: Human Kinetics Publishers, Inc.

Rooney, KJ, RD Herbert and RJ Balnave. 1994. Fatigue contributes to the strength training stimulus. *Medicine and Science in Sports and Exercise* 26 (9): 1160-1164.

Sale, DG. 1988. Neural adaptation to resistance training. *Medicine and Science in Sports and Exercise* 20 (5): S135-S145.

Sanders, MT. 1980. A comparison of two methods of training on the development of muscular strength and endurance. *The Journal of Orthopaedic and Sports Physical Therapy* (spring): 210-213.

Schantz, P, E Randall-Fox, W Hutchison, A Tyden and P-O Astrand. 1983. Muscle fiber type distribution, muscle cross-sectional area and maximal voluntary strength in humans. *Acta Physiologica Scandinavica* 117 (2): 219-226.

Scrimshaw, NS, and VR Young. 1976. The requirements of human nutrition. *Scientific American* 235 (3): 50-64.

Seliger, V, L Dolejs and V Karas. 1980. A dynamometric comparison of maximum eccentric, concentric and isometric contractions using EMG and energy expenditure measurements. *European Journal of Applied Physiology* 45 (2-3): 235-244.

Selye, H. 1956. *The stress of life*. New York, NY: McGraw-Hill.

Sharkey, BJ. 1975. *Physiology and physical activity*. New York, NY: Harper & Row.

_____. 1984. *Physiology of fitness*. Champaign, IL: Human Kinetics Publishers, Inc.

Silver, MD. 2001. Use of ergogenic aids by athletes. *Journal of the American Academy of Orthopaedic Surgeons* 9 (1): 61-70.

Singh, A, FM Moses and PA Deuster. 1992. Chronic multivitamin-mineral supplementation does not enhance physical performance. *Medicine and Science in Sports and Exercise* 24 (6): 726-732.

Skinner, JS. 1995. Understanding the physiological basis of cardiorespiratory fitness. In *The Stairmaster fitness handbook, 2d ed*, ed. JA Peterson and CX Bryant, 57-65. St. Louis, MO: Wellness Bookshelf.

Smith, NJ. 1984. Nutrition. In *Sports medicine*, ed. RH Strauss, 468-480. Philadelphia, PA: W. B. Saunders Company.

Song, TM, L Perusse, RM Malina and C Bouchard. 1994. Twin resemblance in somatotype and comparisons with other twin studies. *Human Biology* 66 (3): 453-464.

Sparling, P, R Recker and T Lambrinides. 1994. Position statement to football players from Cincinnati Bengals Training Staff and nutrition consultant.

Spriet, LL. 1995. Caffeine and performance. *International Journal of Sports Nutrition* 5 (supplement): S84-S99.

St. Jeor, ST, BV Howard, TE Prewitt, V Bovee, T Bazzarre and RH Eckel. 2001. Dietary protein and weight reduction. *Circulation* 104 (15): 1869-1874.

Steinhaus, AH. 1933. Chronic effects of exercise. *Physiological Reviews* 13 (1): 103-147.

Strauss, RH, ed. 1984. *Sports medicine*. Philadelphia, PA: W. B. Saunders Company.

Stromme, SB, and H Skard. 1980. *Physical fitness and fitness testing*. Sandnes, Norway: Jonas Oglaend A.s.

Swanger, T, M Bradley and S Murray. 1996. *Army strength & conditioning manual*. West Point, NY: United States Military Academy.

Taubes, G. 2002. What if it's all been a big fat lie? *The New York Times Magazine*. (July 6): 22-27.

Taylor, MR. 1993. *The dietary supplement debate of 1993: an FDA perspective*. Presented at the Federation of American Societies for Experimental Biology Annual Meeting. New Orleans, LA.

Telford, R, E Catchpole, V Deakin, A Hahn and A Plank. 1992. The effect of 7 to 8 months of vitamin/mineral supplementation on athletic performance. *International Journal of Sports Nutrition* 2 (2): 135-153.

Terjung, RL, P Clarkson, ER Eichner, PL Greenhaff, PJ Hespel, RG Israel, WJ Kraemer, RA Meyer, LL Spriet, MA Tarnopolsky, AJM Wagenmakers and MH Williams. 2000. The ACSM roundtable on the physiological and health effects of oral creatine supplementation. *Medicine and Science in Sports and Exercise* 32 (3): 706-717.

Thacker, SB, J Gilchrist, DF Stroup and CD Kimsey Jr. 2004. The impact of stretching on sports injury risk: a systemic review of the literature. *Medicine and Science in Sports and Exercise* 36 (3): 371-378.

Thompson, CW. 1985. *Manual of structural kinesiology. 10th ed*. St. Louis, MO: Times Mirror/Mosby College Publishing.

Thrash, K, and B Kelly. 1987. Flexibility and strength training. *The Journal of Applied Sport Science Research* 1 (4): 74-75.

Todd, T. 1986. A brief history of resistance exercise. In *Getting stronger, revised ed*, by B. Pearl and G. T. Moran, 413-431. Bolinas, CA: Shelter Publications, Inc.

U. S. Department of Health and Human Services and U. S. Department of Agriculture. 2005. *Dietary guidelines for Americans. 6th ed*. Washington, DC: U. S. Government Printing Office.

Vander, AJ, JH Sherman and DS Luciano. 1975. *Human physiology: the mechanisms of body function. 2d ed*. New York, NY: McGraw-Hill, Inc.

Vanderburgh, PM, and WJ Considine. 1995. Assessing health-related & functional fitness. In *The Stairmaster fitness handbook, 2d ed*, ed. JA Peterson and CX Bryant, 131-156. St. Louis, MO: Wellness Bookshelf.

Wateska, M, and M Bradley. 1998. *Cardinal conditioning*. Palo Alto, CA: Stanford University.

Weight, LM, TD Noakes, D Labadorios, J Graves, D Haem, P Jacobs and P Berman. 1988. Vitamin and mineral status of trained athletes including the effects of supplementation. *American Journal of Clinical Nutrition* 47 (2): 186-191.

Weiss, LW, HD Coney and FC Clark. 1999. Differential functional adaptations to short-term, low-, moderate-, and high repetition weight training. *Journal of Strength and Conditioning Research* 13 (3): 236-241.

Wenger, HA, and GJ Bell. 1986. The interactions of intensity, frequency and duration of exercise training in altering cardiorespiratory fitness. *Sports Medicine* 3 (5): 346-356.

Westcott, WL. 1983. *Strength fitness: physiological principles and training techniques. Expanded ed*. Boston: Allyn and Bacon, Inc.

_____. 1996. *Building strength and stamina: new Nautilus training for total fitness*. Champaign, IL: Human Kinetics.

_____. 1986. Integration of strength, endurance and skill training. *Scholastic Coach* 55 (May/June): 74.

_____. 1989. Strength training research: sets and repetitions. *Scholastic Coach* 58 (May/June): 98-100.

Westcott, WL, and JR Parziale. 1997. Golf power. *Fitness Management* 13 (December): 39-41.

Westcott, WL, RA Winett, ES Anderson, JR Wojcik, RLR Loud, E Cleggett and S Glover. 2001. Effects of regular and slow speed resistance training on muscle strength. *The Journal of Sports Medicine and Physical Fitness* 41 (2): 154-158.

Wilcox, AR. 1990. Caffeine and endurance performance. *Sports Science Exchange* 3 (26): 1-4.

Williams, MH. 1992. *Nutrition for fitness and sport*. Dubuque, IA: Brown & Benchmark.

Williams, MH, and JD Branch. 1998. Creatine supplementation and exercise performance: an update. *Journal of the American College of Nutrition* 17 (3): 216-234.

Willis, T, and KA Beals. 2000. The Zone Diet vs. traditional weight loss diet: effects on weight loss and blood lipid levels. *Journal of the American Dietetic Association* (supplement) 100 (9): A-74.

Wilmore, JH. 1982. *Training for sport and activity: the physiological basis of the conditioning process. 2d ed*. Boston, MA: Allyn and Bacon, Inc.

_____. 1974. Alterations in strength, body composition and anthropometric measurements consequent to a 10-week weight training program. *Medicine and Science in Sports* 6 (2): 133-138.

Winett, RA. 1996. Dose-response. *Master Trainer* 6 (June): 1-2.

Winter, DA. 1990. *The biomechanics of human movement*. New York, NY: Wiley & Sons.

Wirhed, R. 1984. *Athletic ability: the anatomy of winning*. New York: Harmony Books.

Wolf, MD. 1982. Muscles: structure, function and control. In *Strength training by the experts, 2d ed*, by DP Riley, 27-40. West Point, NY: Leisure Press.

Young, WB, and GE Bilby. 1993. The effect of voluntary effort to influence speed of contraction on strength, muscular power, and hypertrophy development. *Journal of Strength and Conditioning Research* 7 (3): 172-178.

About the Author

MATT BRZYCKI, B. S., is the Coordinator of Recreational Fitness and Wellness Programming at Princeton University in Princeton, New Jersey. He has more than 22 years of experience at the collegiate level as a coach, instructor and administrator. His current responsibilities at Princeton University include managing the Stephens Fitness Center and teaching a variety of fitness classes such as Adult Fitness, Introduction to Free Weights, Introductory Strength Training and Women-n-Weights.

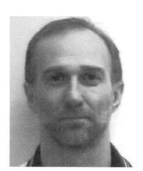

Mr. Brzycki earned his Bachelor of Science degree in health and physical education from Penn State in 1983. He represented the university for two years in the Pennsylvania State Collegiate Powerlifting Championships and was also a place-winner in his first bodybuilding competition. Prior to entering college, he served in the United States Marine Corps from 1975-79 which included a 12-month tour of duty as a Drill Instructor.

He has been a featured speaker at local, regional, state and national conferences, clinics and camps throughout the United States and Canada. This includes presentations at the U. S. Secret Service Academy; the Princeton University Strength & Speed Camp; the National Strength & Science Seminar; the American College of Sports Medicine's Health & Fitness Summit & Exposition; the Tampa Bay Buccaneer Strength and Conditioning Seminar; and the Toronto Football Clinic. He and Stuart Meyers (president of Operational Tactics, Inc.) developed a SWAT (Special Weapons and Tactics) Fitness Specialist Certification Program and they teach the two-day course to law-enforcement personnel. Mr. Brzycki has written more than 260 articles/columns on strength and fitness that have been featured in 40 different publications. He has authored, co-authored or edited 12 other books.

Mr. Brzycki was elected to serve on the Alumni Society Board of Directors for the College of Health & Human Development (Penn State). He was appointed by the governor to serve on the New Jersey Council of Physical Fitness and Sports as well as the New Jersey Obesity Prevention Task Force.